Local Anaesthesia in Dentistry

Jacques A. Baart
Henk S. Brand

Editors

Local Anaesthesia in Dentistry

Second Edition

Editors
Jacques A. Baart
Vrije University Medical Center
Amsterdam, The Netherlands

Henk S. Brand
Academic Centre for Dentistry Amsterdam
Amsterdam, The Netherlands

This work has been first published in 2013 by Bohn Stafleu van Loghum, The Netherlands with the following title: Lokale anesthesie in de tandheelkunde; tweede, herziene druk.

The first edition of the English language edition was first published in 2008 by Wiley-Blackwell with the following title: Local Anaesthesia in Dentistry.

ISBN 978-3-319-43704-0   ISBN 978-3-319-43705-7   (eBook)
DOI 10.1007/978-3-319-43705-7

Library of Congress Control Number: 2017937372

Printed on acid-free paper

This Springer imprint is published by Springer Nature
The registered company is Springer International Publishing AG
The registered company address is: Gewerbestrasse 11, 6330 Cham, Switzerland

This book is dedicated to the memory
of Theo van Eijden en Frans Frankenmolen

Foreword

Patients in current dental care expect painless treatment. To this end, local anaesthesia is the key factor. Modern local anaesthetics are very efficient and safe drugs, and the great majority of patients will not encounter unpleasant side effects nor lasting local or systemic complications. The history of local anaesthesia goes back more than a century, and yet further developments in biological insight and clinical management are still ongoing.

This second edition of *Local Anaesthesia in Dentistry* has been written primarily for dental students, and as such, it covers basic knowledge and recent achievements alike. The editors have produced a balanced composition of essentials within pain physiology, neuroanatomy, pharmacology, aspects related to equipment and techniques for anaesthetising the regions of the oral cavity, local and systemic adverse events, special considerations in children, etc.

Improvements in this second edition of the English version include 45 more pages with new illustrations, a chapter on computer-assisted local anaesthesia, more boxes to emphasise facts, and much more.

The book was originally written and edited in Dutch by Dr. Baart and Dr. Brand. Like the translation of the first edition, the written English is flowing in an easy-to-read style with highlights in boxes and photographic and artistic figures of excellent quality.

The editors must be complimented for the success of an affordable, well-written, and edited textbook to provide theoretical background and practical guidance for dental students in the essentials of local anaesthesia. Also dental practitioners may benefit from the book to bring them on level with current standards.

Søren Hillerup DDS, PhD, Dr Odont
Professor Em., Maxillofacial Surgery
Copenhagen 2017

Contents

Contributors

J.K.M. Aps
University of Washington
Department of Oral Medicine
Seattle, USA
johan.apsdmfr@hotmail.com

J.A. Baart
Academic Centre for Dentistry Amsterdam/
Vrije Universiteit Medical Centre
Department of Oral and Maxillofacial Surgery
Amsterdam, The Netherlands
ja.baart@vumc.nl

L.H.D.J. Booij
Radboud University Medical Centre Nijmegen
Department of Anaesthesiology
Nijmegen, The Netherlands
lhdj.booij@upc.mail.nl

J.F.L. Bosgra
Tergooi hospital, Department of Oral and
Maxillofacial Surgery
Hilversum, The Netherlands
jflbosgra@hotmail.com

H.S. Brand
Academic Centre for Dentistry Amsterdam
Department of Oral Biochemistry
Amsterdam, The Netherlands
hbrand@acta.nl

W.G. Brands
Royal Dutch Dental Association
Nieuwegein, The Netherlands
wbrands1@kpnmail.nl

F.W.A. Frankenmolen[†]
Paediatric Dental Centre
Beuningen, The Netherlands

A.L. Frankhuijzen
Vrije Universiteit Medical Centre
Department of Pharmacology
Amsterdam, The Netherlands
bram.ank@zonnet.nl

G.E.J. Langenbach
Academic Centre for Dentistry Amsterdam
Department of Functional Anatomy
Amsterdam, The Netherlands
g.langenbach@acta.nl

H.P. van den Akker
Academic Centre for Dentistry Amsterdam/
Academic Medical Centre
Department of Oral and Maxillofacial Surgery
Amsterdam, The Netherlands
hpvandenakker@gmail.com

T.M.G.J. van Eijden[†]
Academic Centre for Dentistry Amsterdam
Department of Functional Anatomy
Amsterdam, The Netherlands

[†]Authors were deceased at the time of publication.

Introduction: A Short History of Local Anaesthesia

General anaesthesia already existed before local anaesthesia became available. Actually, general anaesthesia was introduced by the American dentist Horace Wells. In 1844, together with his wife Elizabeth, he witnessed a demonstration whereby the circus owner Colton intoxicated a number of volunteers with laughing gas. One of the volunteers hit himself hard on a chair but did not even grimace. Horace Wells noticed this and concluded that a patient, having inhaled laughing gas, might be able to undergo an extraction without pain. A few days later, Wells took the experiment upon himself and asked a colleague to extract one of his molars after he had inhaled some laughing gas. It was a success. Wells independently organised some additional extraction sessions, after which the Massachusetts General Hospital invited him for a demonstration. This demonstration turned out to be a fiasco. The patient was insufficiently anaesthetised since not enough laughing gas was administered. Wells' life, which had initially been so successful, became a disaster. The physician Morton, a previous assistant to Wells, absconded with the idea of general anaesthesia, but used ether instead of laughing gas for a 'painless sleep'. Morton denied in every possible way that he had stolen the idea from Wells. Wells was greatly incensed by this. Furthermore, Wells was no longer able to practise as a dentist. He became a tradesman of canaries and domestic products and became addicted to sniffing ether. Eventually he was imprisoned for throwing sulphuric acid over some ladies of easy virtue. At the age of 33 years, he made an end to his life in prison by cutting his femoral artery.

The discovery of local anaesthesia is a very different story. One of the first to gain experience with this form of anaesthesia was Sigmund Freud, in 1884. Freud experimented with the use of cocaine. Cocaine had been used for several centuries by the Incas in Peru to increase their stamina. Freud used cocaine in the treatment of some of his patients and then became addicted himself. The German surgeon August Bier observed a demonstration in 1891, whereby the internist Quincke injected – for diagnostic purposes – a cocaine solution into a patient's epidural area, thus anaesthetising and paralysing the legs. Bier took this discovery to his clinic in Kiel and decided to try the technique first on himself and only thereafter to operate on patients under local anaesthesia. Together with his colleague, senior doctor Hildebrandt, he decided to perform an experiment. Bier volunteered to be the guinea pig, and Hildebrandt administered a spinal injection to his boss. This failed, however, due to the fact that the syringe containing the cocaine solution did not fit the needle so a lot of liquor leaked through the needle. It was then Hildebrandt's turn as the test subject, and Bier succeeded in administering an epidural anaesthesia with a cocaine solution. After a few minutes Hildebrandt reported that his leg muscles were numb and his legs were tingling. Bier tested the efficacy of the local anaesthesia by sticking a large injection needle deep into Hildebrandt's upper leg. Hildebrandt did not feel a thing, even when Bier hit his femur skin hard with a wooden hammer. After 45 min, the local anaesthetic began to wear off. The gentlemen then went out for dinner and enjoyed cognacs and good cigars. The next morning, however, the local and systemic disadvantages of this local anaesthesia came to light. Bier had a raging headache after his failed anaesthetic, which lasted 1 week and would only go away if he lay down. Nevertheless, he continued to operate. Hildebrandt was in worse shape. The next day he called in sick; he felt dizzy and was vomiting continually. Walking was difficult, partly because of haemorrhages in his upper and lower leg. On the basis of all these disadvantages, Bier concluded that he would refrain from treating his patients under local anaesthesia. Later, Bier strayed from regular medicine and became an alternative medicine fanatic. However, Bier's extensive observations and descriptions of his experiments with local anaesthesia did not go unnoticed.

In 1899, the French surgeon Tuffer was unaware of Bier's work but operated on a young lady with a hip sarcoma under local anaesthesia, applying a cocaine solution to the spinal canal. Several years later, he operated on patients under local anaesthesia in the kidney, stomach, and even the thoracic wall. The first use of local anaesthesia in dentistry is attributed to the American Halsted, who anaesthetised himself with a cocaine solution.

Because of the high toxicity and addictive effects of cocaine, a safer local anaesthetic was sought. This was eventually found in 1905 in the form of procaine, an ester derivative of cocaine. Procaine became known under the brand name of Novocaine ('the new cocaine'). This remedy was used for many years, but after a while, a stronger anaesthetic was needed. During the Second World War, the Swedish scientist Nils Lofgren succeeded in making the amide compound lidocaine. Lidocaine remedy works faster and more effectively than cocaine and is not addictive. However, how to administer the local anaesthetic remained a problem. In 1947, the American company Novocol marketed the cartridge syringe, glass cartridges with local anaesthetic and disposable needles. With this, modern local anaesthesia was born. Lidocaine and articaine, which was introduced in the 1970s, are now the most commonly used local anaesthetics in dentistry.

J.A. Baart
J.F.L. Bosgra

Further Reading

1. Bennion E. Antique dental instruments. London: Sotheby's Publications; 1986.
2. Richards JM. Who is who in architecture, from 1400 to the present day. London: Weidefeld and Nicolson; 1977.
3. Sydow FW. Geschichte der Lokal- und Leitungsanaesthesie. In: Zinganell K, editor. Anaesthesie – historisch gesehen. Berlin/Heidelberg: Springer; 1987.

Pain and Impulse Conduction

L.H.D.J. Booij

© Springer International Publishing Switzerland 2017
J.A. Baart, H.S. Brand (eds.), *Local Anaesthesia in Dentistry*, DOI 10.1007/978-3-319-43705-7_1

According to the World Health Organization, pain is defined as an 'unpleasant sensation that occurs from imminent tissue damage'. From a physiological perspective, pain is a warning system. During dental treatment, patients will experience pain as something unpleasant. Pain will also make it impossible for the dentist to work accurately.

1.1   Pain Receptors

Pain stimuli are primarily generated by the relatively amorph sensory nerve endings of the Aδ and C fibres. These free nerve endings (nociceptors; see ◘ Fig. 1.1) are sensitive to a variety of mechanical, thermal and chemical stimuli and are therefore called polymodal. Nociceptors do not display adaptation: nociceptive responses will occur as long as the stimulus is present. Nociceptors have a high threshold for activation, so only potentially noxious stimuli are detected. The detection of the stimulus is performed by the receptors, present on the sensory nerve endings. They consist of ion channels that respond to mechanical stimulation, temperature or chemical substances. The conversion of the stimulus into an electric signal is called transduction.

During tissue damage, several substances are released that are able to stimulate the nociceptors, such as histamine, serotonin, bradykinin, prostaglandin E_2 and interleukins. These substances activate the nociceptors and reduce their threshold (sensitisation). There is also feedback regulation from the central nervous system. Once pain has been observed, the receptors become more sensitive for nociceptive stimuli. This mechanism plays a role in the development of chronic pain.

Nociceptors are also present in the teeth and the oral cavity and are usually sensitive to a specific neurotransmitter. Important are the fluid-filled canals in the dentine, where free endings of the trigeminal nerve are present which are able to register pressure changes in the canals. Odontoblasts may play an additional role by releasing calcium and ATP. This ATP stimulates the endings of the trigeminal nerve. The sensory nervous system also contains 'physiological' sensors. These are small end organs of the sensory nerves, such as the Krause, Meissner and Pacini bodies (see ◘ Fig. 1.2). These 'physiological' sensors usually only respond to one specific stimulus (warmth, touch, smell, etc.) and are, as such, unimodal. Besides this, they exhibit the phenomenon of adaptation; the response to a stimulus disappears during prolonged or persistent stimulation. In the case of excessive stimulation, these 'physiological' sensors may also initiate pain sensation. Transduction occurs in ion channels.

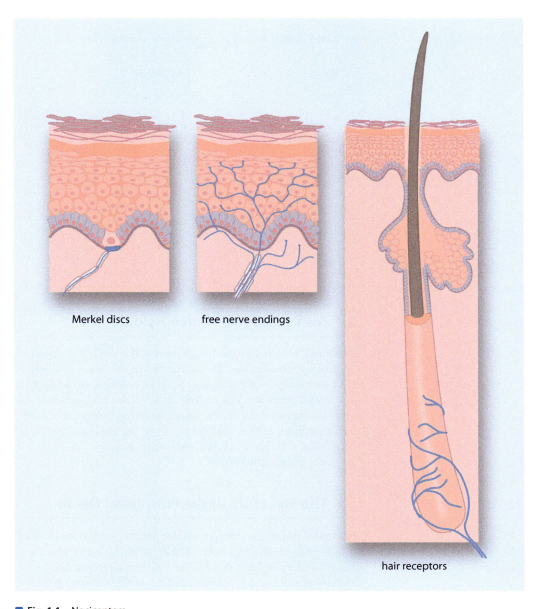

Merkel discs   free nerve endings

hair receptors

■ **Fig. 1.1**   Nociceptors

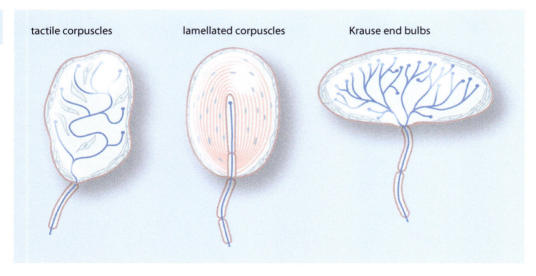

tactile corpuscles   lamellated corpuscles   Krause end bulbs

◘ Fig 1.2 Physiological sensors

1.2   Nerve Impulse Transmission

The stimuli, received by the nociceptors and converted into nerve impulses, eventually must be interpreted in the brain. The nerve impulse is transported within the sensory nervous system, wherein three nerve fibres are successively linked. The first nerve fibres form the peripheral nerve. The second and third are present in the central nervous system and form nerve bundles (pathways or tracts). The cell nuclei of the individual neurons are grouped together in ganglia and nuclei.

1.2.1   The Structure of the Peripheral Nerve

Nociceptive stimuli are transported along sensory thinly myelinated Aδ and unmyelinated C fibres. Other types of nerve fibres are involved in the transport of other sensory stimuli (see ◘ Box 1.1).

A peripheral nerve is composed of nerve fibres from a group of neurons, enwrapped in a connective tissue network. The individual fibres may, or may be not, surrounded by an isolating myelin layer, Schwann's sheath.

The cell body is the metabolic centre of the neuron (◘ Fig. 1.4) where most cell organelles are produced. Dendrites transport impulses towards the cell body and axons transmit signals away from the cell body. Some axons are surrounded by a myelin sheath, while others are not. The axons and dendrites are elongated and form the nerve fibres. At the end of the dendrites, receptors are present that can receive signals. At the end of the axons are synapses, where the impulse is transmitted to another nerve cell or to a cell of the end organ.

Box 1.1   Nociceptive Pathways

There are several types of peripheral nerve fibres in the body. Nociceptive stimuli are received by nociceptors and then propagated via an A or C fibre (Fig. 1.3). The first are thinly myelinated with a fast conduction of stimuli (1.2–40 m/s), whereas the second are unmyelinated with a slow conduction (0.13–1.2 m/s). The A fibres have different subtypes: α, β, γ and δ.

The C fibres conduct impulses generated by temperature, mechanical and chemical stimulation. The Aα fibres conduct motor impulses for the body's posture and movement (proprioception); the Aβ fibres transport impulses generated by touch and signals from the skin mechanoreceptors. The Aγ fibres are involved in the regulation of the muscular tone, and the Aδ fibres conduct pain impulses and temperature signals.

The cell bodies of these primary neurons are located in the dorsal root ganglion and, for the face, in the nuclei of the trigeminal nerve. The axons run through Lissauer's tract to the dorsal horn of the spinal cord, where they connect to the secondary sensory neuron in Rexed's laminae. This secondary sensory neuron crosses the midline and ascends as the spinothalamic tract. The spinothalamic tract forms synapses with nuclei of the thalamus, where it projects onto the somatosensory cortex. Descending pathways from the somatosensory cortex modulate the nociceptive system. From these fibres, the neurotransmitters serotonin and noradrenalin are released. Also the secondary neuron of the trigeminal nerves crosses the midline and projects to the cortex through the thalamus.

axon type	Aα	Aβ	Aδ	C
diameter (µm)	13-20	6-12	1-5	0,2-1,5
speed (m/s)	18-120	35-75	5-35	0,5-2,0

▢ Fig. 1.3   Primary afferent axons

dendrites

cell body

node of Ranvier

myelin
sheath

Schwann cell

synapse

■ Fig. 1.4 The nerve cell

Nerves are bundles of nerve fibres held together by connective tissue (■ Fig. 1.5). In addition, each individual axon is also surrounded by connective tissue (endoneurium). Bundles of nerve fibres form a fascicle, which is also held together by connective tissue (perineurium). A number of fascicles are held together again by connective tissue (epineurium), forming a nerve.

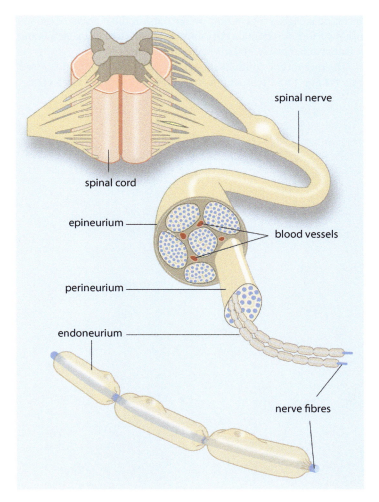

spinal nerve

spinal cord

epineurium

blood vessels

perineurium

endoneurium

nerve fibres

◼ Fig. 1.5 The peripheral nerve

1.2.2 Impulse Formation

The generation and conduction of impulses in nerve fibres is a complicated process. In order to excite electrical impulses, a change in electrical charge must take place.

Cells are surrounded by a semipermeable membrane that is only permeable to water. A selective ion pump actively pumps potassium ions into the cell and sodium ions out of the cell. This results in a concentration gradient of sodium and potassium ions over the membrane. The cell cytoplasm contains a high concentration of negatively charged proteins, which give the cell a negative charge compared with its environment. Extracellularly, negatively charged ions are also present, primarily chloride ions. On both sides of the membrane, the electrical charge is balanced by positively charged ions (sodium, potassium, calcium). Because the concentration of anions on the inside is slightly higher than on the outside, the number of cations inside will therefore be higher than outside. This causes a transmembrane potential difference of −60 mV, called the resting potential.

The membrane contains ion channels with an open and closed state (■ Fig. 1.6). These channels can be activated by an electrical

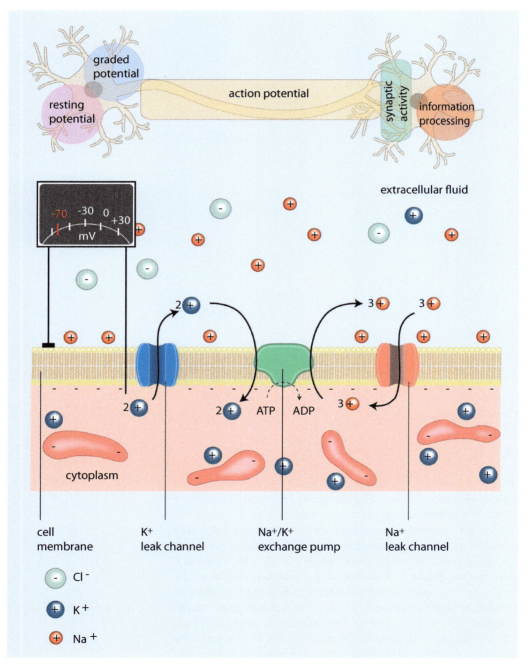

■ **Fig. 1.6** Semipermeable membrane with ion channels

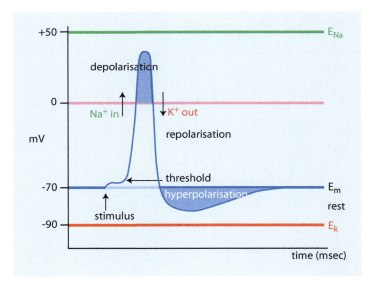

◘ **Fig. 1.7** The action potential

stimulus ('voltage gated'), by a chemical stimulus ('ligand gated') or by a mechanical stimulus (see ◘ Box 1.2). When ion channels are open, ions move along the concentration gradient. At rest, primarily potassium channels are open, so that potassium ions try to leave the cell. However, the relative overload of anions in the cell (proteins) counteracts the outflow of cations. When the sodium channels of the membrane open, sodium ions will move in: in other words, the membrane has a hole.

The inflow of sodium ions distorts the electrical equilibrium, so that a local depolarisation occurs and potassium ions can leave the cell. This restores the balance between anions and cations (repolarisation). During the depolarisation and the beginning of the repolarisation, no new depolarisation can occur (refractory period).

When the local depolarisation is slight, the equilibrium is quickly restored (◘ Fig. 1.7). Only when the local

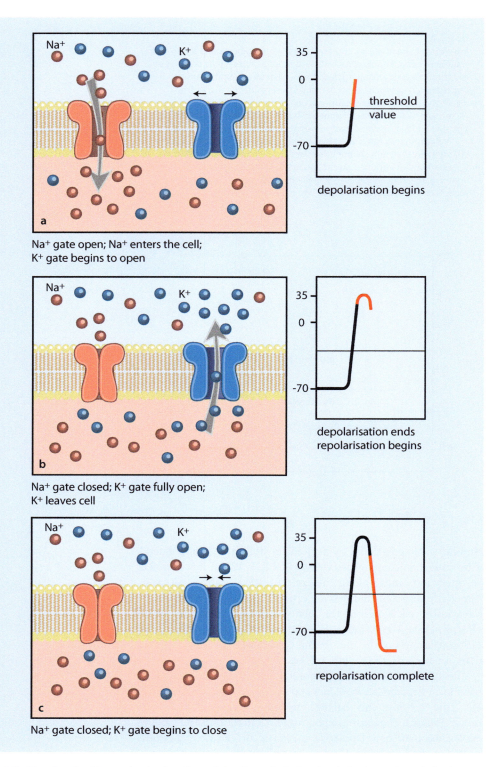

■ **Fig. 1.8**   Transfer of sodium and potassium through ionchannels during depolarisation and repolarisation

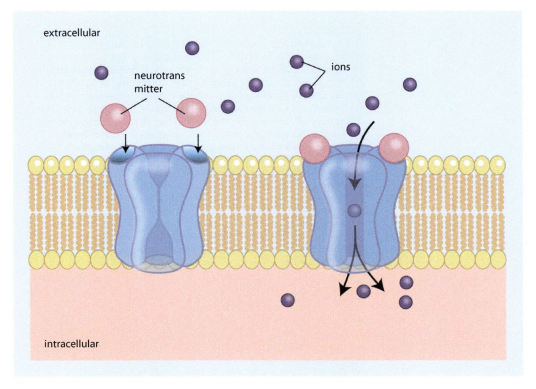

extracellular

neurotrans
mitter

ions

intracellular

◻ **Fig. 1.9**   Activation of a ligand-gated ionchannel

depolarisation reaches a certain threshold value (approx. −50 mV) does an action potential appear. Thus, there is an 'all-or-none' effect.

The height of the threshold value, necessary for an action potential to develop, is determined by factors such as the duration and strength of the depolarising stimulus and the status of the receptor. Through this, the voltage-gated sodium channels are opened, so that an influx of sodium occurs and the membrane polarity reverses.

The sodium channels remain open only for approx. one millisecond, after which they close again. The potassium channels are then still open, and the outflow of potassium through voltage-gated potassium channels restores the electrical equilibrium, and even hyperpolarisation takes place. Then, the voltage-gated potassium channels close and the sodium-potassium pump restores the starting situation. The number of sodium and potassium ions that has to be moved in order to generate an action potential is very small.

1

Box 1.3
The motoric and sensory innervation of the face is segregated, in contrast to the other parts of the human body. The face is motoric innervated by the facial nerve (n. VII) and sensory innervated by the trigeminal nerve (n. V). Exceptions are the motoric fibres of the mandibular nerve that innervate the masticatory muscles and the sensoric fibres of the facial nerve that ensure the perception of taste, as long as this comprises the anterior two-thirds of the tongue. The motoric branch of the mandibular nerve ramifies from the other parts very early, and subsequently this branch is not anaesthetised during blockade of the inferior alveolar nerve and the lingual nerve. The motoric branches to the mylohyoid muscle and the anterior part of the digastric muscle are affected by mandibular block anaesthesia, but the practical consequences are limited. Regional block anaesthesia only affects the function of a nerve distally from the location where the anaesthetic has been applied. Therefore, during dental treatment, pain will not be observed, but the patient will still be able to use the facial and masticatory muscles (◘ see Fig. 2.8).

Box 1.4
In practice, the lower lip often slightly droops after anaesthesia of the inferior alveolar nerve, despite that the motoric innervation is not provided by this nerve. Probably the drooping is caused by anaesthesia of muscle spindles of the orbicularis oris muscle, thereby reducing the basal tonus of the lower lip muscle at the anaesthetised side.

Box 1.5
Local anaesthetics administered to tissues will be absorbed in the bloodstream. The rate of absorption is dependent on the blood flow in the tissue, the concentration of the anaesthetic and the administered amount. If an overdose of anaesthetic is administered or the anaesthetic is injected into a blood vessel, the blood concentration may become too high. This will affect the amygdala and/or heart muscle. This may cause an 'epileptic insult', usually followed by unconsciousness as first the inhibitory tonus of the central nervous system is inhibited and only thereafter the stimulatory impulses. The impaired conduction of impulses within the heart may result in a decreased heart rate or even a cardiac arrest.

1.2.3 Impulse Conduction and Transfer

Once a stimulus is converted into an action potential, the action potential must be propagated along the nerve. This occurs through sequential depolarisations along the membrane, which are initiated by the activation of fast sodium channels.

In myelinated nerves, sodium channels are only present at the gaps in the myelin sheath, the nodes of Ranvier, which causes a jumping (saltatory) conduction (◘ Fig. 1.10a). In unmyelinated

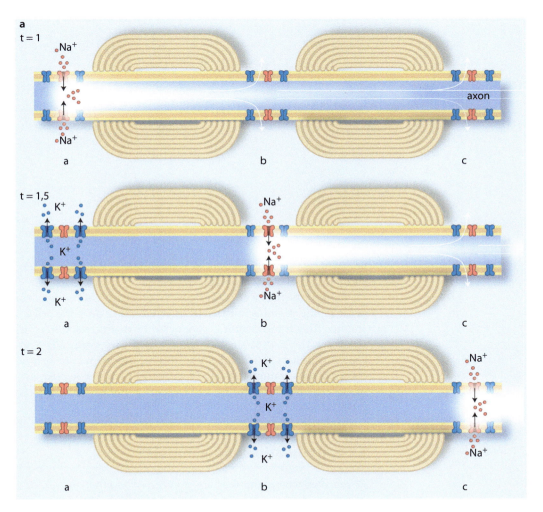

◘ **Fig. 1.10**　**a** Saltatory conduction. **b** Continuous conduction

1

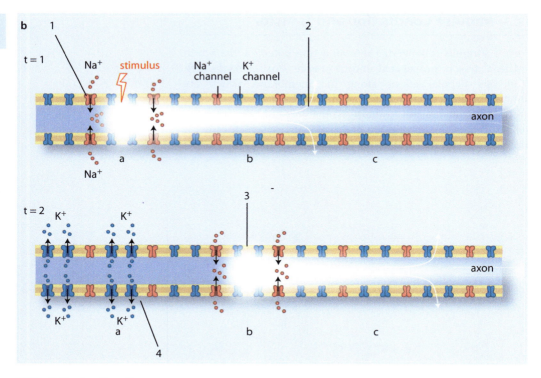

Fig. 1.10   (continued)

nerve fibres, the conduction is a continuous process over the entire length of the neuron (■ Fig. 1.10b).

Because the sensory nervous system consists of three successive neurons, the stimulus must be transferred from one nerve cell to another. This transmission is conducted by neurotransmitters in synapses. The neurotransmitter is released presynaptically and activates postsynaptic receptors. These postsynaptic receptors consist of ion channels that open once activated, which depolarises the cell membrane, creating an electrical stimulus again, that is propagated along the nerve fibre.

1.2.4 Modulation of the Impulse

At the sites where impulses are transferred to other nerves, the impulse stimulus can be enhanced or subdued. This process is called neuromodulation. This can occur both peripherally as well as at connection points in the central nervous system.

One of the most frequent forms of neuromodulation is that affecting the voltage-gated sodium channels involved in the formation and conduction of action potentials. Excitatory neurotransmitters lower the resting potential (hypopolarisation). Consequently, the threshold level can be reached more easily, through which an action potential can occur more quickly. Inhibitory transmitters will only cause an opening of potassium channels, which induces hyperpolarisation of the membrane and an action potential will develop less easily. These mechanisms affect the transmission of impulses. The release of neurotransmitters can also be influenced by presynaptic receptors. Many receptors are involved in these systems, usually selective ion channels (see ◼ Box 1.6).

Modulation of impulse conduction can also happen through cellular second messengers. An example of this is prostaglandin E_2, which is released during tissue damage. Prostaglandin E_2 increases the sensory transduction via a G protein (protein kinase A). This facilitates the inflow of sodium and the outflow of potassium, changing the electrical charge over the membrane; thus, the nerve cell will be stimulated more easily. As a result, a nociceptive stimulus will be propagated more easily. There is, therefore, a local amplification system. On the other hand, afferent fibres exist that have a subduing effect on transduction. For example, activation of μ-receptors (opioids) increases the stimulus threshold which negatively modulates transmission.

Box 1.6 Modulation of Nociceptive Stimuli

Various ion channels are involved in the modulation of nociceptive stimuli. They are present, among other places, in the peripheral endings involved in the stimulus perception where they modulate the sensitivity: temperature-sensitive ion channels (vanilloid receptors, VR1), acid-sensitive channels (proton activated receptors) and purine-sensitive ion channels (P2X receptors). Besides these, there are also voltage-gated receptors that especially allow passage of sodium or potassium ions and ligand-gated channels that primarily affect the release of neurotransmitters.

The neurotransmitters are released from the presynaptic nerve ending in large amounts and are able to change the polarity of nerve membranes by opening ion channels. This creates a postsynaptic potential that, depending on the nature, causes either a depolarisation (excitatory postsynaptic potential) or a hyperpolarisation (inhibitory postsynaptic potential). When neurotransmitters open cation channels, the nerve is excited (depolarisation). When they open anion channels, inhibition occurs (hyperpolarisation). The most important excitatory neurotransmitter in the nociceptors is glutamate. Substance P plays an important role in peptidergic fibres. Neuropeptides not only have a role in modulating the input to spinal nociceptive neurons and autonomic ganglia but also cause vasodilation, contraction of smooth muscles, release of histamine from mast cells, chemoattraction of neutrophil granulocytes and proliferation of T lymphocytes and fibroblasts.

1

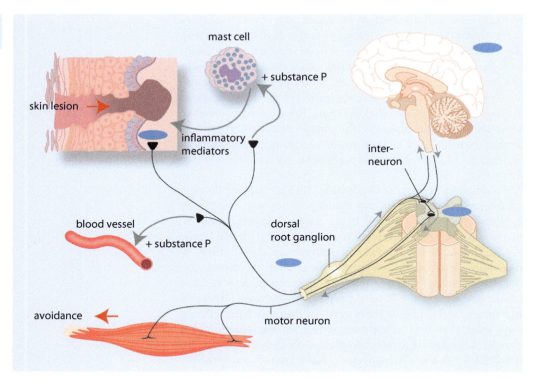

mast cell

+ substance P

skin lesion

inflammatory
mediators

inter-
neuron

blood vessel

+ substance P

dorsal
root ganglion

avoidance

motor neuron

Fig. 1.11   Intervention sites for analgesics

Pharmacological treatment of pain often intervenes in these modulation systems (■ Fig. 1.11).

1.3   Perception of Pain

Consciousness is a requisite of the perception of pain. Ultimately, the nociceptive stimuli reach the primary sensory cortex, whereby pain is experienced and a physiological response is induced. Pain leads to the release of hormones, such as cortisol and catecholamines, which stimulate the catabolism. Respiration frequency and the speed of blood circulation also increase. Fear and emotion are caused by the transfer of the stimulus to the limbic system.

There are great differences in pain perception between men and women. Women have a lower pain threshold and a lower tolerance for nociceptive stimuli than men. Furthermore, there are great sociocultural differences in the sensation of pain: one patient may experience no pain, while another may cry out from pain, though stimulated by the same stimulus. The emotional state of the patient and environmental factors play an important role in the experience of pain. Fear and excitement have a large influence on the individual pain experience. Fear mobilises the body to take action in order to avoid or reduce impending damage. As a result, fear causes hypoalgesia. Excitement has the opposite effect.

Aromas have a great impact on mood; this influence is much greater than that of music, which is often used in dental practices. Additionally, the effect of aromas takes place much faster than that of sound or visual stimuli. It has recently been shown that scents, by a change in mood, indeed have a fast and positive influence on the experience of pain. Here, there still seems to be a role for the dentist.

1.4   Nociception in the Orofacial Area

The process of transduction, transmission, modulation and perception also occurs in the head and neck area. Tooth pain is caused by stimulation of the polymodal nociceptors in the dental pulp and dentine that respond to mechanical and thermal activation. They can also react to pressure. The intensity of the pain is determined by the frequency of the sensory stimulation and by the number of nerve fibres that are excited. Temperature stimulations induce immediate pain responses through the Aδ fibres. When a tooth is stimulated mechanically, fluid moves in the pulp and the channels in the dentine, which alters the form of the nerve membrane and a stimulus is excited slowly (via C fibres). After application of something cold, the stimulus extinguishes after a while, because vasoconstriction induces lack of oxygen in the nerve. Electrical stimulation induces ion transport, resulting in the stimulation of nerve endings. The same process occurs in osmotic stimulation, for example, by sugar and salt. Chemical inflammatory mediators cause the stimulation of nociceptors on the C fibres in the pulp. Substance P, calcitonin gene-related peptide and neurokinin A have been found in the periodontium and in the pulp of teeth. In painful teeth, the concentration of these inflammatory mediators is increased. They are released from the nerve fibre endings during stimulation and activate the nociceptors. The stimuli are thus propagated by primary Aδ and C fibres, primarily in the trigeminal nerve. At the Gasserian ganglion, they synapse onto secondary fibres that run to the brainstem trigeminal nuclei. From there, they project to the thalamus and the cerebral cortex.

The secondary C fibres end in the most caudal part of the ventrobasal thalamus, run from there to the intralaminar nucleus of the thalamus (forming the activating part of the reticular formation) and project to the cerebral cortex and the hypothalamus. The secondary Aδ fibres terminate in the caudal nucleus, where they activate pain tracts to the most caudal part of the ventrobasal thalamus. From there tertiary tracts run to other parts of the thalamus and somatosensory cortex.

Anatomy of the Trigeminal Nerve

T.M.G.J. van Eijden and G.E.J. Langenbach

© Springer International Publishing Switzerland 2017
J.A. Baart, H.S. Brand (eds.), *Local Anaesthesia in Dentistry*, DOI 10.1007/978-3-319-43705-7_2

The trigeminal nerve is the fifth cranial nerve (n. V), which plays an important role in the innervation of the head and neck area, together with other cranial and spinal nerves. Knowledge of the nerve's anatomy is very important for the correct application of local anaesthetics.

2.1   Introduction

The trigeminal nerve contains a large number of sensory (afferent) and motor (efferent) neurons. The sensory fibres carry nerve impulses towards the central nervous system, while the motor fibres carry impulses away from the central nervous system. The trigeminal nerve has a wide innervation area (◘ Fig. 2.1). The nerve provides the sensitivity of the dentition, the mucosa of the mouth, nose and paranasal sinuses and the facial skin. The nerve also contains motor fibres that innervate, among others, the masticatory muscles. Although the trigeminal nerve is the most important nerve for the sensory and motor innervation of the oral system, the facial (n. VII), glossopharyngeal (n. IX), vagus (n. X) and hypoglossal (n. XII) nerves are also of significance. The n. VII, n. IX and n. X, for example, take care of the taste sense, and the n. IX and n. X provide the general sensation (pain, touch and temperature) of

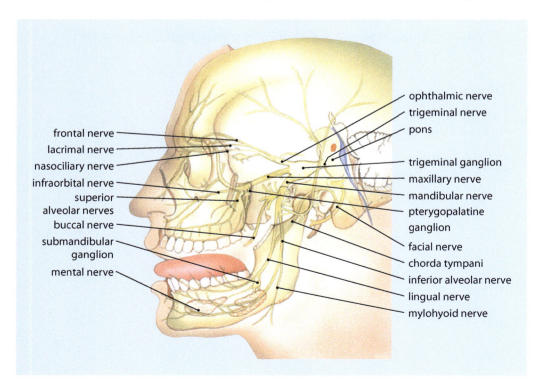

◘ **Fig. 2.1**   Overview of the trigeminal nerve (lateral view)

the pharynx, soft palate and the back of the tongue, while the n. XII is responsible for the motor innervation of the tongue. Although these latter nerves do play an important role in innervating the oral cavity, they will only be mentioned marginally in this book.

2.2   The Central Part of the Trigeminal Nerve

2.2.1 Origin

The trigeminal nerve emerges from the middle of the pons, at the lateral surface of the brainstem. The nerve consists of two parts here: the sensory fibres form a thick root and the motor fibres form the much thinner motor root. These two roots run to the front of the petrous part of the temporal bone where the large sensory trigeminal ganglion (semilunar or Gasserian ganglion) lies in a shallow groove surrounded by dura mater.

The trigeminal ganglion is formed by the aggregation of cell bodies of sensory neurons. After the ganglion, three branches of the trigeminal nerve can be distinguished: the ophthalmic nerve (n. V_1), the maxillary nerve (n. V_2) and the mandibular nerve (n. V_3). The motor root joins the mandibular nerve only, once it has exited the skull via the foramen ovale. The sensory areas covered by the three main branches are generally as follows:

- The ophthalmic nerve carries sensory information from the skin of the forehead, the upper eyelids and the nose ridge and the mucosa of the nasal septum and some paranasal sinuses.
- The maxillary nerve innervates the skin of the middle facial area, the side of the nose and the lower eyelids, the maxillary dentition, the mucosa of the upper lip, the palate, the nasal conchae and the maxillary sinus.
- The mandibular nerve innervates the skin of the lower facial area, the mandibular dentition, the mucosa of the lower lip, cheeks and floor of the mouth, part of the tongue and part of the external ear.

Of all the areas that the trigeminal nerve innervates, the oral cavity is the most enriched with sensory neurons. The density of sensory neurons in the mouth is much larger than in any other area, e.g. the facial skin. This density of sensory neurons increases from the back to the frontal area of the mouth.

Most of the trigeminal ganglion neurons are pseudo-unipolar. This means that each neuron in the ganglion has a peripheral and a central process. The peripheral process (axon) is relatively long and carries the impulses coming from sensory receptors (◼ Box 2.1). The central process (dendrite) is short and enters the pons and synapses with the sensory trigeminal nucleus situated in the

Box 2.1 Receptors

Sensory nerves are capable of picking up impulses from the external world and the body. The ends of the fibres themselves function as receptors, or there are special receptors (e.g. taste receptors, muscle spindles). Each receptor type is the most sensitive to one specific sensation. There are, for example, mechanoreceptors (reacting to touch and mild pressure), thermoreceptors (reacting to temperature) and nociceptors (reacting to tissue damage). Nociceptors serve pain sensation. There are also so-called proprioceptors. These are mostly found in muscles (muscle spindles and Golgi tendon organs) and in the joint capsules. They supply information on the position of the jaw and the speed and direction of movement. This form of sensation is called proprioceptive sensibility or proprioception.

There are a great number of receptors present in the facial skin and lips, in the mucosa of the oral cavity and tongue, in the teeth and the periodontium and in the masticatory muscles and temporomandibular joint.

brainstem. The proprioceptive fibres in the trigeminal ganglion are an exception. Their cell bodies are not situated in this ganglion but in the mesencephalic nucleus of the trigeminal nerve. The proprioceptive fibres are found in the motor root of the trigeminal nerve and carry impulses from, among others, muscle spindles of the masticatory muscles.

The trigeminal ganglion has somatotopy. This means that the neurons in the ganglion are arranged in the same order as the areas that are innervated by the three main branches of the trigeminal nerve. The cell bodies of the ophthalmic nerve are grouped medially in the ganglion, while those of the mandibular nerve are grouped laterally. In the middle of these two groups, the cell bodies of the maxillary nerve can be found.

2.2.2 Trigeminal Nuclei

The trigeminal nerve has a sensory and motor nucleus within the brainstem (◘ Fig. 2.2). The sensory nucleus lies laterally, and most of the sensory neurons of the trigeminal nerve contact (synapse) with the neurons in this nucleus. The nucleus forms a long column that extends from the midbrain to the spinal cord. It consists of (from cranial to caudal) the mesencephalic, the principal and the spinal trigeminal nuclei.

Proprioceptive information from, for example, the masticatory muscles is managed in the mesencephalic nucleus. The principal trigeminal nucleus mainly receives touch and pressure impulses from the entire oral area, whereas the spinal trigeminal nucleus

mesencephalon
cranial nerve IV
sensory root

ophthalmic nerve
trigeminal ganglion
maxillary nerve
mandibular nerve
motor root
pons

cranial
nerve VI up to XII

medulla oblongata

mesencephalic nucleus
of trigeminal nerve

motor nucleus of
trigeminal nerve

proprius nucleus
of trigeminal nerve

spinal tract nucleus
of trigeminal nerve

🔲 **Fig. 2.2**   The motor and sensory nuclei in the brainstem (medial view). The sensory nuclei are shown in *blue* and the motor nuclei in *red*

receives information on pain, temperature and pressure from the entire trigeminal area. All information received via the sensory trigeminal nuclei is managed and integrated in, among others, the thalamus via ascending paths. After this the information is brought to various areas of the cerebral cortex, where perception occurs.

The motor neurons of the trigeminal nerve are grouped in a motor nucleus that lies medially to the sensory nucleus in the centre of the pons. The axons of these motor neurons run to (among others) the masticatory muscles. As previously described, these axons pass the trigeminal ganglion as an independent bundle (motor root), without synapsing within it. Similar to the motor neurons in the spinal column, the motor neurons in the motor trigeminal nucleus are directly stimulated via the corticobulbar tract, originating from the contralateral cerebral cortex. Within the motor nucleus, there is a large amount of somatotopy, i.e. the motor neurons that innervate (parts of) the different muscles are grouped together. Via fibres coming from the sensory mesencephalic nucleus, the motor trigeminal nucleus receives proprioceptive information from the masticatory muscles, temporomandibular joint and periodontium.

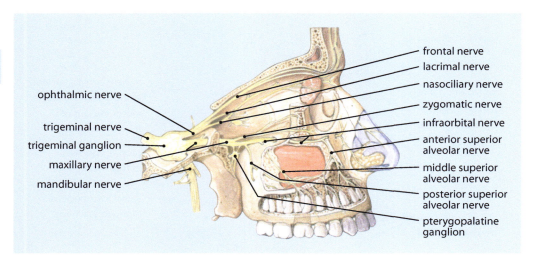

ophthalmic nerve

trigeminal nerve
trigeminal ganglion
maxillary nerve
mandibular nerve

frontal nerve
lacrimal nerve
nasociliary nerve
zygomatic nerve
infraorbital nerve
anterior superior alveolar nerve
middle superior alveolar nerve
posterior superior alveolar nerve
pterygopalatine ganglion

◼ **Fig. 2.3**   The branching of the ophthalmic and maxillary nerves (lateral view)

2.3   The Peripheral Part of the Trigeminal Nerve

2.3.1 Ophthalmic Nerve

The ophthalmic nerve (n. V$_1$) enters the cranial part of the orbit (◼ Fig. 2.3). This nerve carries only sensory fibres, and, just before leaving the cranial cavity through the superior orbital fissure, it branches off into three: the nasociliary, frontal and lacrimal nerves. These nerves run in the roof of the orbit and are involved in the sensory innervation of a large number of structures, such as the mucosa of the frontal, sphenoid and ethmoid sinus, the mucosa of the nasal cavity and nasal septum, the skin of the nose ridge, the upper eyelid and forehead till the hairline and the mucosa that covers the eyeball and inside of the eyelids.

2.3.2 Maxillary Nerve

The maxillary nerve (n. V$_2$), too, is solely sensory. It enters the pterygopalatine fossa (▶ see Sect. 2.4.1) via the foramen rotundum (◼ Fig. 2.3). Through the inferior orbital fissure, it reaches the floor of the orbit and proceeds there as the infraorbital nerve, first in the infraorbital sulcus and then in the infraorbital canal. It then reaches the face via the infraorbital foramen.

Within the pterygopalatine fossa, the maxillary nerve is connected via a number of branches to the upper side of the parasympathetic pterygopalatine ganglion. Sensory fibres run through these branches which exit on the lower side of the

Fig. 2.4 The maxillary nerve (medial view)

Fig. 2.5 The path of the nasopalatine nerve along the nasal septum

ganglion (Figs. 2.4 and 2.5) and form, among others, the following nerves:

- The nasal nerves and nasopalatine nerve that run through the sphenopalatine foramen to the nasal mucosa. The nasal nerves innervate the back part of the nasal mucosa. The nasopalatine nerve, which runs forwards along the nasal septum and reaches the oral cavity through the incisive canal, innervates the mucosa and bone of the nasal septum, frontal two-thirds of the palate and the palatal gingiva of the maxillary teeth.
- The greater palatine nerve that runs via the greater palatine canal to the mucosa of the hard palate where it subsequently innervates the palatal gingiva of the maxillary alveolar process and the pulp of the palatal first molar and premolar.

2

— The lesser palatine nerves that run to the mucosa of the soft palate via the lesser palatine canals.

Together with the palatine nerves, there are also parasympathetic and orthosympathetic fibres that run from the pterygopalatine ganglion to the salivary glands in the palatal mucosa.

In the pterygopalatine fossa, the maxillary nerve also branches into the posterior superior alveolar nerve and the zygomatic nerve (◘ Fig. 2.3). The posterior superior alveolar nerve exits the pterygopalatine fossa through the pterygomaxillary fissure and runs over the maxillary tuberosity. The nerve divides into a large number of little branches, the posterior superior alveolar rami, which enter the wall of the maxilla through small openings and innervate the maxillary molars and corresponding buccal gingiva. The zygomatic nerve arrives in the orbit via the inferior orbital fissure and branches into the zygomaticotemporal and zygomaticofacial nerves. These exit the lateral orbital wall through small canals in the zygomatic bone and innervate the skin above. The zygomatic nerve also contains postganglionic parasympathetic fibres that come from the pterygopalatine ganglion and that join the lacrimal nerve (branch of n. V_1) for the lacrimal gland.

As it runs along the orbital floor, the infraorbital nerve branches in two: the middle superior alveolar nerve, for the innervation of the maxillary premolars and the corresponding buccal gingiva, and the anterior superior alveolar nerve, for the maxillary canine and incisors and the corresponding buccal gingiva. These nerves usually run between the mucosa and outer wall of the maxillary sinus. There they divide into a number of small branches, the medial and anterior superior alveolar rami that penetrate into the maxillary alveolar process via small openings. Inside the bone, they form together with the posterior superior alveolar rami, right above the apices, an extensive nervous network – the superior alveolar plexus – from which short little branches are sent to the dentition and gingiva.

Once the infraorbital nerve reaches the face via the infraorbital foramen, it splits into a large number of branches for the sensory innervation of the skin of the lower eyelid (palpebral rami), the infraorbital region, the side of the nose (nasal rami) and the skin and mucosa of the upper lip (labial rami).

2.3.3 **Mandibular Nerve**

The mandibular nerve (n. V_3) contains both sensory and motor fibres. This nerve exits the skull through the foramen ovale and ends in the infratemporal fossa (▶ see Sect. 2.4.2; ◘ Fig. 2.6). The mandibular nerve is located just below this foramen between the

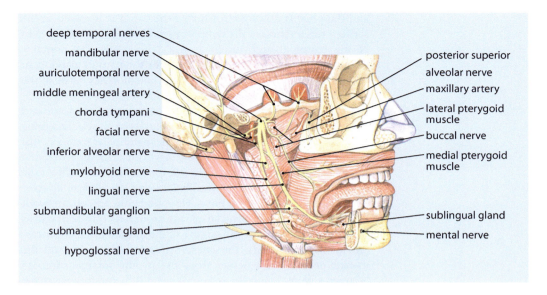

deep temporal nerves

mandibular nerve

auriculotemporal nerve

middle meningeal artery

chorda tympani

facial nerve

inferior alveolar nerve

mylohyoid nerve

lingual nerve

submandibular ganglion

submandibular gland

hypoglossal nerve

posterior superior alveolar nerve

maxillary artery

lateral pterygoid muscle

buccal nerve

medial pterygoid muscle

sublingual gland

mental nerve

▪ **Fig. 2.6**   The mandibular nerve (lateral view)

lateral pterygoid muscle and the tensor veli palatini muscle. The nerve sends a motor branch to the latter muscle.

The mandibular nerve splits into two main branches, the anterior and posterior trunks. From the anterior trunk, a sensory nerve emerges, the buccal nerve, and a number of motor nerves, i.e. the pterygoid nerves, the deep temporal nerves and the masseteric nerve. Three branches emerge from the posterior trunk: the auriculotemporal nerve (sensory), the lingual nerve (sensory) and the inferior alveolar nerve (mixed sensory and motor).

The buccal nerve runs along the medial surface of the upper head of the lateral pterygoid muscle and moves laterally between the two heads of the muscle. The nerve contains postganglionic parasympathetic fibres, coming from the otic ganglion, for the salivary glands in the buccal mucosa. The nerve innervates the skin and mucosa of the cheek and the buccal gingiva of the mandibular alveolar process at the level of the molars and premolars. The course of the nerve on the anterior side of the ramus shows a great variation.

The pterygoid nerves are short motor branches for the medial and lateral pterygoid muscles. The masseteric nerve runs laterally along the top of the upper head of the lateral pterygoid muscle and reaches the deep surface of the masseter muscle via the mandibular notch. The deep temporal nerves also run high along the lateral pterygoid muscle and penetrate the medial side of the temporal muscle.

The auriculotemporal nerve arises as two roots encircling the middle meningeal artery. After the roots have merged to a single nerve, this nerve first runs laterally behind the mandibular neck and then bends upwards in front of the ear. It is involved in the sensory innervation of the temporomandibular joint and the skin of the temporal and auricle region. The nerve also contains postganglionic parasympathetic fibres for the parotid gland from the otic ganglion. This parasympathetic ganglion lies between the mandibular nerve and the tensor veli palatini.

At its origin, the inferior alveolar nerve contains motor and sensory fibres. It runs deep to the lateral pterygoid muscle. Emerging from beneath this muscle, it directs to the mandibular foramen. Just before it enters the mandibular canal, it gives off its motor mylohyoid branch for the mylohyoid muscle and for the anterior belly of the digastric muscle. Inside the mandibular canal, the inferior alveolar nerve contains only sensory fibres. Here, under the apices, a network is formed, the inferior alveolar plexus, from which little branches are sent to the dentition and gingiva of the inferior alveolar process ($\blacksquare$ Fig. 2.7). Anteriorly, the inferior alveolar nerve gives off the mental nerve. This emerges from the mental foramen, located between and just below the apices of P_1 and P_{2inf}, and innervates the skin of the chin, the skin and mucosa of the lower lip and the buccal gingiva of the inferior alveolar process at the level of the canine and incisors. The last stretch of the inferior alveolar nerve inside the mandibular canal that runs in the direction of the symphysis is not located in a canal. This part of the inferior alveolar nerve is usually named as a separate nerve, the incisive nerve.

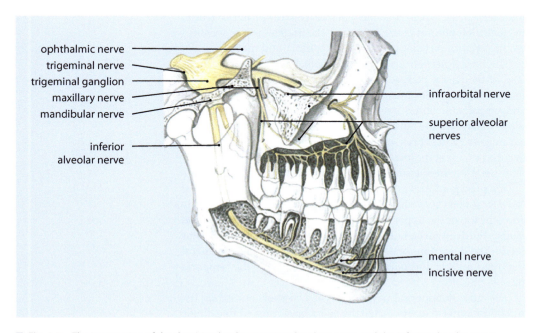

$\blacksquare$ **Fig. 2.7** The innervation of the dentition by the superior alveolar nerves and the inferior alveolar nerve

ophthalmic nerve

maxillary nerve

nerve of
pterygoid canal

pterygopalatine
ganglion

palatine nerves

lateral pterygoid
muscle

tensor veli
palatini muscle

medial pterygoid
muscle

motor root

sensory root

middle meningeal
artery

greater petrosal
nerve

mandibular nerve

facial nerve

otic ganglion

chorda tympani

pterygoid nerve

auriculotemporal
nerve

maxillary nerve

inferior alveolar
nerve

lingual nerve

mylohyoid nerve

external carotid
artery

◘ Fig. 2.8   The mandibular nerve (medial view)

Box 2.2   Innervation of the Tongue
Various nerves are involved in the sensory and motor innervation of the
tongue. The general sensitivity (pain, touch, temperature) of the
anterior two-thirds of the tongue is supplied by the lingual nerve
(branch of the n. V_3). The specific sensitivity (taste) of the anterior
two-thirds is supplied by the chorda tympani (branch of the n. VII) that
has joined with the lingual nerve. The sensitivity, general and specific,
of the posterior third of the tongue is supplied by the glossopharyngeal
nerve (n. IX). The motor innervation of the tongue takes place through
the hypoglossal nerve (n. XII).

The lingual nerve is joined, directly after its separation of n.
V_3, by the chorda tympani (◘ Fig. 2.8). This is a branch of the
facial nerve with preganglionic parasympathetic fibres from the
brainstem and sensory nerves for the taste of the anterior two-
thirds of the tongue (◘ Box 2.2). The lingual nerve runs deep to
the lateral pterygoid muscle and forwards over the lateral surface
of the medial pterygoid muscle. At the level of the apices of the
third mandibular molar, it lies immediately beneath the mucosa

a

b

buccal nerve

superior alveolar nerves

infraorbital nerve

nasopalatine nerve

greater palatine nerve

lesser palatine nerves

buccal nerve

inferior alveolar nerve

mental nerve

lingual nerve

glossopharyngeal nerve

Fig. 2.9 The sensory innervation of the oral cavity. **a** The palate, the superior alveolar process, the cheek and the upper lip. **b** The tongue, the inferior alveolar process, the cheek and the lower lip

against the inner side of the mandible. It continues superiorly to the mylohyoid muscle, passing under the submandibular duct, and then ascends in the tongue. The section of the lingual nerve that comes from n. V_3 supplies the general sensitivity (pain, touch, temperature) of the anterior two-thirds of the tongue, the mucosa of the floor of the mouth and the lingual gingiva of the inferior alveolar process. The submandibular parasympathetic ganglion is closely related to the lingual nerve. This ganglion is connected by a number of small branches to the underside of the nerve. Preganglionic parasympathetic fibres from the chorda tympani reach the ganglion via these branches. The postganglionic parasympathetic fibres run to the submandibular and sublingual glands.

A schematic summary of the sensory innervation of the oral cavity with the areas supplied by the various branches of the maxillary and mandibular nerves is given in **Fig. 2.9**.

2.4   Deep Areas

The pterygopalatine fossa and the infratemporal fossa (including the pterygomandibular space) are deep areas in the head that are of great significance for block anaesthesia of (branches of) the maxillary and mandibular nerves, respectively.

2.4.1 Pterygopalatine Fossa

The pterygopalatine fossa is a small pyramid-shaped space that lies medially to the infratemporal fossa. The tip of the pyramid is directed downwards. The fossa is found behind the orbit and the maxillary tuberosity and also lateral to the posterior part of the nasal cavity. The posterior wall is formed by the pterygoid process of the sphenoid bone, the medial wall by the perpendicular plate of the palatine bone and the anterior wall by the maxillary tuberosity.

The pterygopalatine fossa has a large number of openings and forms an important junction for blood vessels and nerves. In the top of the fossa, the cranial cavity can be accessed posteriorly via the foramen rotundum, and it is connected anteriorly via the medial part of the inferior orbital fissure to the orbit. Laterally the infratemporal fossa can be reached via the triangular pterygomaxillary fissure. Medially the sphenopalatine foramen forms the connection with the nasal cavity. The downward-directed tip of the fossa runs narrowly to the greater palatine canals, thus reaching the palate.

The maxillary artery reaches the pterygopalatine fossa through the pterygomaxillary fissure. Within the fossa, the artery gives off various branches:

- The posterior superior alveolar artery and the infraorbital artery that run alongside the veins and nerves of the same name.
- The descending palatine artery that runs downwards through the greater palatine canal and splits into the greater palatine artery and the lesser palatine arteries. The greater palatine artery runs forwards over the hard palate, whereas the lesser palatine arteries serve the soft palate (❑ Fig. 2.10).
- The sphenopalatine artery that runs through the sphenopalatine foramen to the mucosa of the nasal cavity.

Veins, which drain regions supplied by these arteries, connect with the pterygoid plexus. This area can be approached by an injection dorsolateral of the M_{2sup} with the needle point directed medially. Aspiration is essential.

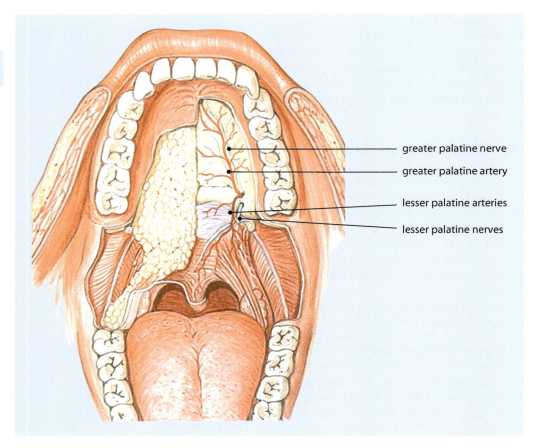

greater palatine nerve

greater palatine artery

lesser palatine arteries

lesser palatine nerves

■ Fig. 2.10   The palate from below

As mentioned previously, the maxillary nerve enters the pterygopalatine fossa via the foramen rotundum. The nerve runs forwards along the top side of the fossa and enters the orbit via the inferior orbital fissure. From this point, the nerve is called the infraorbital nerve. In the fossa, the maxillary nerve gives off the posterior superior alveolar nerve that leaves the fossa through the pterygomaxillary fissure and uses the surface of the maxillary tuberosity to reach the maxillary molars. Immediately beneath the maxillary nerve lies the pterygopalatine ganglion, which serves the parasympathetic innervation of, among others, the lacrimal gland, salivary glands of the palate and mucous glands in the nasal cavity, using the various branches of the maxillary nerve. The orthosympathetic innervation of these structures originates from the superior cervical ganglion which branches into a network around the arteries of the head region. The maxillary nerve also branches off caudally in the greater and lesser palatine nerves for the sensory innervation of the hard and soft palate, respectively; they leave the pterygopalatine fossa via the greater palatine foramen and the lesser palatine foramina. Ventrally and medially, the maxillary nerve branches off into the nasopalatine nerve, for the innervation of the nasal cavity via the sphenopalatine foramen. This nerve eventually also reaches the anterior part of the palate via the nasal septum and the incisive canal.

2.4.2 Infratemporal Fossa and Pterygomandibular Space

The infratemporal fossa is an area on the inner side of the zygomatic arch and the mandibular ramus. The other bony boundaries of the fossa are the greater wing of the sphenoid bone on the upper side, the maxillary tuberosity on the anterior side and the lateral plate of the pterygoid process (sphenoid bone) on the medial side. The pharynx wall provides a soft tissue boundary, medially and ventrally.

On the posterior side, the infratemporal fossa changes, without a clear border, into the parapharyngeal and retropharyngeal space. Medially the fossa provides access to the pterygopalatine fossa via the pterygomaxillary fissure. The fossa is connected via the foramen ovale and the foramen spinosum to the cranial cavity, and via the lateral part of the inferior orbital fissure, it is connected to the orbit.

The lateral pterygoid muscle and the medial pterygoid muscle are situated within this fossa (■ Fig. 2.11). Besides these muscles, the infratemporal fossa is filled to a large extent by a fat body that

■ **Fig. 2.11**   The infratemporal fossa viewed from behind

parotid gland
external carotid artery
retromandibular vein
facial nerve
mandibular ramus
inferior alveolar artery, vein and nerve
pterygomandibular space
masseter muscle
medial pterygoid muscle
pharynx
buccinator muscle

Fig. 2.12   Horizontal cross-section of the oral cavity and of the pterygomandibular space

is an extenuation of the buccal fat pad (of Bichat). Blood vessels and nerves are embedded within this fat, i.e. the maxillary artery, the pterygoid venous plexus and branches of the mandibular nerve.

The lateral and medial pterygoid muscles, together with the mandibular ramus, border a separate space within the infratemporal fossa, the so-called pterygomandibular space. In a frontal cross-section, the pterygomandibular space is triangular in shape (resembling a paper cornet), enclosed medially by the medial pterygoid muscle, cranially by the lateral pterygoid muscle and laterally by the mandibular ramus. The space is bordered ventrally by the pharynx wall and dorsally by the deep section of the parotid gland (**Fig. 2.12**). The space merges into the submandibular space ventro-caudally, and more medially and caudo-cranially, it merges into the parapharyngeal and retropharyngeal spaces, which eventually convert into the mediastinum and the pericard.

The most important artery in the infratemporal fossa is the maxillary artery (**Fig. 2.13**). This artery supplies blood to the nasal cavity, the palate, the maxilla and mandible and the masticatory muscles. The artery enters the fossa between the mandibular neck and the sphenomandibular ligament. It subsequently runs to the lower margin of the lateral pterygoid muscle and continues medially or laterally from this muscle to the pterygopalatine fossa. Besides

□ Fig. 2.13 The maxillary artery (lateral view)

giving off a large number of branches to masticatory muscles (masseteric artery, deep temporal arteries, pterygoid arteries), the maxillary artery also branches off, among others, the middle meningeal artery, which reaches the cranial cavity via the foramen spinosum, and the inferior alveolar artery. The latter nerve enters, together with the inferior alveolar vein and nerve, the mandibular canal via the mandibular foramen and supplies blood to the lower jaw. The mental artery, which branches off from the inferior alveolar artery at the end of the mandibular canal, exits with the mental vein and nerve through the mental foramen and supplies blood to the chin and lower lip. Within the infratemporal fossa, the veins continue to follow the path of the arteries. These veins lead into the extensive pterygoid venous plexus, which lies laterally of the lateral pterygoid muscle. The pterygoid plexus connects posteriorly, via the short maxillary vein, with the retromandibular vein and anteriorly with the facial vein.

The mandibular nerve reaches the infratemporal fossa via the foramen ovale. The parasympathetic otic ganglion, which innervates, among others, the parotid gland and the salivary glands in the cheek, lies directly under the foramen ovale, on the medial side of the nerve. This nerve initially runs between the medial side of the lateral pterygoid muscle and the medial pterygoid muscle and gives off motor branches here for the innervation of the lateral and medial pterygoid muscles (pterygoid nerves), the temporalis muscle (deep temporal nerves), the masseter muscle (masseteric nerve) and the tensor tympani and tensor veli palatini muscles. Sensory branches are the buccal, lingual, inferior alveolar and auriculotemporal nerves. The buccal nerve runs laterally between the two heads of the lateral pterygoid muscle and then continues to the cheek. This nerve also contains parasympathetic fibres for the innervation of the salivary glands. The auriculotemporal nerve initially consists of two roots, which pass around the medial meningeal artery. The auriculotemporal nerve runs in a dorsolateral direction to the mandibular neck, continues behind it and innervates, among others, the temporomandibular joint, the skin behind this joint and the skin in front of the ear. This nerve also contains parasympathetic fibres for the parotid gland, which originate from the otic ganglion. The two largest branches of the mandibular nerve are the inferior alveolar nerve and the lingual nerve. These two nerves initially run medially from the lateral pterygoid muscle. On the medial side of this muscle, the chorda tympani also joins the lingual nerve. The two nerves enter the pterygomandibular space at the lower margin of the lateral pterygoid muscle.

Pharmacology of Local Anaesthetics

A.L. Frankhuijzen

© Springer International Publishing Switzerland 2017
J.A. Baart, H.S. Brand (eds.), *Local Anaesthesia in Dentistry*, DOI 10.1007/978-3-319-43705-7_3

Local anaesthetics are the most commonly used pharmaceuticals in dentistry. When used at the recommended doses, they interfere reversibly with the generation of the action potential and with cellular impulse conduction by blockading the sodium channels in the nerve cell. This results in a local insensibility to pain stimuli.

3.1   Classification

Local anaesthetics share several common characteristics in their molecular structure (■ Fig. 3.1). A lipophilic group can be identified which determines the lipid solubility. Another part contains a hydrophilic group that determines the degree of water solubility. Usually the lipophilic part of the molecule is an aromatic structure that contains a benzene ring. The hydrophilic part contains a secondary or a tertiary amine. Both parts are present at the opposite ends of the molecule and connected by an intermediate section. This intermediate section consists of an ester or an amide group and a relatively short chain of four to five carbon atoms (■ Box 3.1).

In other words, local anaesthetics can be classified according to their molecular structure into two classes: the (amino-) esters and the (amino-) amides. Both groups differ in the way in which they are metabolised.

In the ester anaesthetics, the aromatic part containing the benzene ring is derived from para-amino benzoic acid (PABA).

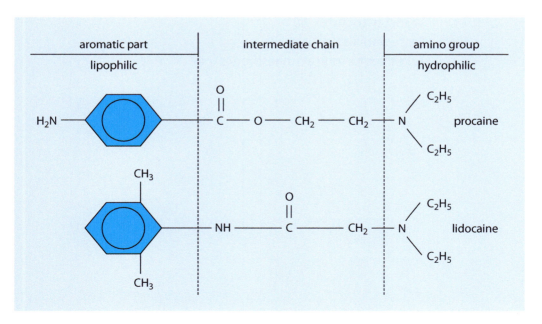

■ **Fig. 3.1**   Molecular structure of an ester-linked (procaine) and amide-linked local anaesthetic (lidocaine) (Modified from Borchard (1985) Aktuelle Aspekte der Zahnärzlichen Lokalanästhesie, Hoechst AG)

Box 3.1
In general, carbon groups can be added to each of the three parts of the molecule (up to a certain maximum). These alterations in molecular structure result in local anaesthetics with strongly different pharmacokinetic properties, since this changes the degree of protein binding, the lipid solubility and the way the local anaesthetic is eliminated. This may result in large differences in onset time, duration of action and effectiveness of local anaesthesia (◨ Table 3.1).

◨ **Table 3.1** An overview of regularly used local anaesthetics with average values of onset time, duration of action and effectiveness relative to prilocaine

	Onset of action after	Duration of action	Effectiveness
Articaine	5 min	1–3 h	3
Bupivacaine	8 min	3–7 h	16
Lidocaine	5 min	½–2 h	4
Mepivacaine	4 min	1–2 h	2
Prilocaine	3 min	2–2½ h	1

The data presented have only meaning for comparison purposes. In the dental practice, these factors strongly depend on the location and method of administration

The intermediate chain, characteristic for this group, contains an ester binding (see ◨ Fig. 3.1). Well-known examples of an ester-type anaesthetic are procaine and tetracaine.

Amide-type anaesthetics have been developed more recently and are characterised by the presence of an amide binding in the intermediate chain, as in lidocaine (see ◨ Fig. 3.1). The amides can further be divided into three subgroups: xylidines, toluidines and thiophenes. Xylidines are tertiary amines with an aromatic part that contains two methyl groups. Representatives from this group are lidocaine (Xylocaine®), mepivacaine (Scandicaine®) and bupivacaine (Marcaine®) (◨ Box 3.2).

Box 3.2
The tertiary amine part of mepivacaine contains a piperidine ring with a methyl group attached, instead of two methyl groups. Bupivacaine also contains a piperidine ring but with a butyl group attached. This butyl group is responsible for the stronger local anaesthetic effect of bupivacaine and the very long duration of action of this local anaesthetic (◨ Table 3.1).

In toluidines, the benzene ring contains a single methyl group and the amine part contains a secondary amine. A frequently used local anaesthetic from this group is prilocaine (Citanest®).

Thiophenes, like articaine (Ultracain®, Septanest®), have a slightly different molecular structure. They contain a sulphur ring in the aromatic part of the molecule. This is probably the reason why this local anaesthetic has a better penetration into the mucosa and the jaw bone.

3.2   Pharmacodynamics

Local anaesthetics differ considerably in onset time, duration of action and strength of the analgesic effect. The strength of the local anaesthetic effect is directly related to the lipid solubility of the local anaesthetic.

Of the series bupivacaine – articaine – lidocaine – prilocaine – mepivacaine, the first anaesthetic is the most lipid soluble and the last one the least. The same order applies to the strength of the analgesic effect of these compounds (◘ Box 3.3). The differences in analgesic strength effect of the compounds, however, seem smaller than theoretically expected (see ◘ Table 3.1). Probably, pharmacokinetic aspects are also important for the strength of the analgesic effect. An overview of factors that can affect the intrinsic activity of local anaesthetics is presented in ◘ Table 3.2.

> **Box 3.3**
> The potency of a local anaesthetic is expressed by the parameter C_m, defined as the minimum concentration of local anaesthetic required to reduce the amplitude of the action potential by 50 % within 5 min in a solution with pH 7.2–7.4 and a stimulus frequency of 30 Hz. Of course, this parameter can only be determined with in vitro experiments.

3.3   Pharmacokinetics

3.3.1 Physical-Chemical Characteristics

Local anaesthetics are weak bases, unstable and poorly water soluble. With a single exception, they are tertiary amines.

□ **Table 3.2** Some factors that affect the intrinsic properties of local anaesthetics	
Factor	**Mechanism**
Pregnancy	Progesterone can potentiate the nerve-blocking effect of the local anaesthetic
pH alteration	Inflammation and uraemia lower the tissue pH. This reduces the percentage of the neutral base form. A pH alteration can also affect the binding to plasma and tissue proteins and seems relevant for the rapid appearance of tolerance during a repeat injection
Vasodilatation	Intrinsic vasodilatation causes rapid elimination from the area of injection. For example, bupivacaine is a vasodilator
Vasoconstriction	A vasoconstrictor masks the inherent vasodilatory properties of the local anaesthetic and causes an increased effect that also lasts longer

Therefore, hydrochloric acid (HCl) is added to the local anaesthetic, which converts the tertiary amine, expressed below as R_3N, into a chloride salt:

$$R_3N + HCl \rightarrow R_3NH^+ + Cl^-$$

This increases the stability and water solubility of a local anaesthetic:

$$R_3NH^+ + H_2O \overset{K_a}{\leftrightarrow} R_3N + H_3O^+$$

R_3NH^+ represents the water-soluble, ionised quaternary cation form of the local anaesthetic, which is responsible for the analgesic effect. This 'active' form is in equilibrium with the 'inactive' form, the uncharged tertiary base R_3N (□ Boxes 3.4 and 3.5). The equilibrium constant K_a of most local anaesthetics is between 7 and 8.

Box 3.4

The relative proportion of the base (R_3N) and cationic form (R_3NH^+) depend on the pK_a (the dissociation constant of the local anaesthetic), the pH of the solution and the pH at the site of injection, as defined by the Henderson-Hasselbalch equation:

$$\log(C_i/C_o) = pK_a - pH$$

In this equation, C_i represents the concentration local anaesthetic in the active, ionised cationic form (R_3NH^+) and C_o the concentration of the inactive, unionised base form (R_3N). When the pH at the site of injection has the same value as the pK_a, 50 % of the local anaesthetic will be present in the unionised form. With a low pH at the injection site, e.g. an injection into inflamed tissue, the percentage of the unionised form will be less than half. Under this condition, less local anaesthetic will be available for diffusion through the lipid membrane to the inside of the nerve cell. This means that the dose administered will analgesically be less effective than assumed based on the dose injected.

The pK_as of some regularly used local anaesthetics are presented in ▫ Table 3.3.

▫ **Table 3.3** A local anaesthetic with a different pK_a or a change in pH affects the percentage of anaesthetic present in the unionised, inactive base form

	pK_a	pH = 7.0	pH = 7.4	pH = 7.8
Articaine	7.8	13	29	50
Bupivacaine	8.1	7	17	33
Lidocaine	7.7	17	33	55

Box 3.5

Local anaesthetics are less effective in inflamed areas. Only the unionised, lipophilic form of a local anaesthetic is able to cross the cell membrane. The addition of HCl results in a solution of local anaesthetic with a pH of 4–6. Due to the presence of these protons, the equilibrium reaction shifts to the right and the ionised form of the local anaesthetic will dominate. After the administration, the buffering capacity of the tissues returns the pH to the normal value of 7.4. At this pH, the equilibrium returns to the left, which increases the concentration of unionised local anaesthetic. The acid environment that occurs in inflamed tissues results in a low tissue pH. Therefore, the local anaesthetic will be present predominantly in the ionised form, which is not able to cross the membrane, and consequently local anaesthetics are less effective in inflamed tissues. In addition, the hyperaemia present in inflamed tissues will carry away the local anaesthetic at an increased rate.

A similar mechanism operates during the administration of a repeat injection of an additional amount of local anaesthetic. When the dentist notices that the anaesthesia is not sufficient, the injection of an additional (large) amount of local anaesthetic will create an acid environment, since the injection fluid itself has a low pH of 4–6.

3.3.2 Diffusion

From the site of administration, a local anaesthetic must cross several barriers to reach the actual site of action. For this, the uncharged base form of the local anaesthetic is necessary (R_3N). This form is lipophilic (fat soluble), enabling it to pass the cell membrane of neurons.

The fat solubility of a local anaesthetic is primarily determined by the charge of the molecule and – to a lesser extent – by the length of the molecule skeleton: the longer the chain, the greater the fat solubility.

Once the uncharged lipophilic form is inside the cell, a new equilibrium with the water-soluble charged form will be established. The intracellular pH is lower than outside, so the equilibrium will shift towards R_3NH^+, the active cationic form of the anaesthetic. Consequently, the proportion between both forms (R_3N and R_3NH^+) plays an essential role in the function of local anaesthetics.

It generally applies that the closer the pK_a value of an anaesthetic to the pH of the injection site, the higher the concentration (C_o) of the uncharged base form (R_3N) of the molecule which is necessary for the diffusion and penetration of the nerve membrane. Choosing a local anaesthetic with a low pK_a or increasing the pH of the local anaesthetic solution will increase the percentage of the lipid-soluble uncharged form of the molecule. This is presented in ◻ Table 3.3, which lists the percentages of uncharged base form of three local anaesthetics at different pHs.

However, for the spread from the administration site to the site of action, a local anaesthetic must have a certain degree of water solubility. For this diffusion in the interstitial fluid between the cells, the water-soluble ionised form (R_3NH^+) is important.

Therefore, both forms of the local anaesthetic, the unionised lipophilic base form (R_3N) and the hydrophilic ionised form (R_3NH^+), must be present in sufficient amounts. This is embedded in their characteristics of being a weak base, where both forms of the local anaesthetic are in equilibrium.

3.3.3 Mode of Action of Local Anaesthetics

Local anaesthetics block the development of an action potential and conduction in the cell membrane. They achieve this by inhibiting the voltage-dependent increase in sodium conductivity over the cell membrane.

It is generally assumed that the most frequently used local anaesthetics act by a combination of membrane expansion and blockade of the sodium channels on the inside of the neuron. The uncharged, lipophilic form of the anaesthetic (R_3N) penetrates the lipid part of the membrane, producing a structural change of the lipid bilayer which disturbs the conduction in the membrane of the neuron. This so-called membrane expansion is responsible for approximately 10 % of the total activity of most local anaesthetics.

The remaining 90 % of the activity depends on an interaction between the charged cationic form of the molecule (R_3NH^+) and the phospholipid phosphatidyl-L-serine in the neuronal membrane. This interaction causes a disturbance of the calcium binding, with the closure of the sodium channel as a result. The strength of the effect of local anaesthetics on sodium channels is dependent on the frequency of the action potential. On one hand, when the sodium channel is open, it is more accessible for the local anaesthetic. On the other hand, local anaesthetics have a higher affinity with open sodium channels.

The total process is called conduction blockade or membrane stabilisation and consists of a decrease in sodium conduction and a reduction of the rate of depolarisation. In addition, the threshold potential level will no longer be reached, so an action potential cannot occur anymore. However, the resting potential, the threshold potential and the repolarisation of the cell membrane will not or hardly be affected.

3.3.4 Protein Binding

Local anaesthetics bind reversibly to both plasma and tissue proteins. They bind primarily to globulins, erythrocytes and less to plasma albumin. Bupivacaine and articaine are strongly bound to plasma proteins (>90 %); mepivacaine, lidocaine and prilocaine are less strongly bound (80, 60 and 55 %, respectively).

The degree of protein binding is a determining factor for the duration time of a local anaesthetic. In general, the higher the degree of binding to plasma proteins, the longer the local anaesthetic will be active. The plasma protein-bound fraction of the local anaesthetic functions as a depot, from which the free local anaesthetic can be released. Remarkably, prilocaine, with a relatively low degree of binding to plasma proteins, binds strongly to tissue proteins, so potentially a toxic concentration will be reached less easily (owing to a larger distribution volume).

3.3.5 Onset Time and Duration of Action

The onset time and the duration of action of local anaesthetics can vary considerably (◘ Box 3.6). In general, the lower the pK_a of a local anaesthetic (or the higher the pH at the injection site), the shorter the onset time. This is a direct result of the increase in the

> **Box 3.6**
> The diameter and myelination varies amongst the different types of nerve fibres, which affects the order in which they are being blocked. After the administration of a local anaesthetic around a peripheral nerve, first stimulus conduction is inhibited in the least myelinated fibres, especially in the preganglionic autonomic B fibres. This inhibits the vasoconstrictive activity of these nerve fibres, resulting in vasodilatation and an increased skin temperature. Next, inhibition of pain and temperature perception will follow, due to blockade of the Aδ and C fibres.
> The function of the Aγ and Aβ fibres – responsible for proprioception and touch and pressure perception – is switched off last of all or, in some cases, remains intact. The latter sometimes induces a very unpleasant sensation in patients. During dental treatment, the patient does not feel pain but will experience the touch of the dentist. In most cases, explanation and information will relieve complaints that may arise from this strange phenomenon. Finally and eventually, the motor Aα fibres are blocked.

concentration of the unionised, lipophilic form of the local anaesthetic (see ◘ Table 3.3). With identical pK_as, the degree of lipid solubility is the determining factor: the higher the lipid solubility, the shorter the onset time.

In addition to the characteristics mentioned above, the total dose (milligrammes) directly determines the onset time (at clinically used dosages). The volume determines the spread. Finally, the concentration determines the strength of the local anaesthetic effect.

The determining factor for the duration of the local analgesic effect is diffusion from the site of administration, followed by redistribution throughout the tissues. In this, the blood flow is the most important factor. Therefore, both the total dose and the lipid solubility and the presence of a vasoconstrictor affect the duration time. Doubling the dose does not increase the duration time by a factor of two, but only by one half-life time. The addition of a vasoconstrictor to the local anaesthetic is the most important factor in increasing the duration time of short- and intermediate-acting local anaesthetics, such as lidocaine and articaine.

3.3.6 Local Elimination

Finally, local anaesthetic is removed from the site of administration by the blood, where the degree of vascularisation of the tissue determines the amount and velocity. Inherent characteristics of the local anaesthetic (such as vasodilatation) and the total injected dose are additional determining factors.

If a local anaesthetic is administered without a vasoconstrictor, it will disappear from the site of administration in three phases.

◻ Table 3.4 Half-life values of the three phases of plasma elimination of local anaesthetics in healthy individuals			
	α-phase (sec)	β-phase (min)	γ-phase (hour)
Articaine	30	102	1.3
Bupivacaine	160	200	3.5
Lidocaine	60	96	1.5
Mepivacaine	40	114	2.0
Prilocaine	29	93	1.2

The initial rapid α-phase represents redistribution by the general circulation from the site of administration to vessel-rich tissues; the slower β-phase represents redistribution to tissues with less blood supply, while the slowest γ-phase represents the metabolism and excretion of the local anaesthetic. In general, these three phases are shorter for high lipophilic and low protein-bound local anaesthetics. ◻ Table 3.4 shows the half-lives of the three phases for some frequently used local anaesthetics. These characteristics also depend on the physical condition of the patient. For example, a patient with heart failure has a slower α- and β-phase and – partly thereby – a slower metabolisation and excretion (γ-phase).

From ◻ Table 3.4 it is clear that prilocaine has the fastest redistribution phases (α- and β-phase) as well as the highest clearance and metabolism in the lungs and kidneys (γ-phase). Furthermore, prilocaine has the lowest inherent vasodilator activity and the lowest binding to plasma proteins, the latter resulting in a large distribution volume. The result of all these factors is that prilocaine is 60 % less toxic than all other local anaesthetics. However, prilocaine has one disadvantage: it is a toluidine derivative, and during degradation of toluidines, the metabolite orthotoluidine is generated. This orthotoluidine can oxidise the Fe^{2+} in haemoglobin to Fe^{3+}, which reduces the oxygen transport capacity, and methaemoglobinaemia develops (see ◻ Box 11.1).

3.3.7 Enhanced Local Elimination

A recent development within local anaesthesia in dentistry is the use of phentolamine. It can be used in case an enhanced elimination of the local anaesthetic after dental treatment is desirable.

After administration of a local anaesthetic, it is possible that soft tissues like cheeks, tongue and lips remain numb for an unwanted period of time, with the concomitant risk of bite wounds. Therefore, it could be beneficial to be able to reduce prolonged numbness in certain patients, to reduce the risk of bite wounds.

> **Box 3.7**
>
> Local anaesthetics are used in dentistry in order to achieve reversible anaesthesia. When used at the recommended doses, they are very safe. However, all local anaesthetics are potentially neurotoxic. In rare cases, a permanent sensibility disorder may occur after the administration of a local anaesthetic, in particular after mandibular block anaesthesia (▶ see Sect. 10.6). The sensibility disorder usually involves the inferior alveolar nerve and the lingual nerve. Possible explanations for such injection-related sensibility disorder are a mechanical trauma of the nerve by the needle and a neurotoxic effect of the anaesthetic on the axon or the myelin sheath of the nerve, or an alteration of the micro-environment of the nerve.
>
> Damage to the axon appears to be the most likely explanation for a permanent neurological defect. The mechanism underlying this is not fully understood. Most likely, the inhibition of the fast axonal transport, in combination with a disruption of the structure of the nerve, results in degeneration of the axon.
>
> When the neurotoxic effect of local anaesthetics should have a common origin, the incidence of sensitivity disorders should not to be related to local anaesthetic used. However, recent retrospective studies of permanent sensibility in the United States, Canada and Denmark reported that the number of cases of permanent paraesthesia when using 4 % articaine were about five times higher than expected, based on the market share of this anaesthetic. In the United States and Canada, 4 % prilocaine caused more frequently sensitivity disorders than local anaesthetics used at lower concentrations. These studies suggest that the neurotoxicity of local anaesthetics used at a 4 % solution is higher than that of local anaesthetics at lower concentrations.

In the United States, phentolamine is available to reduce anaesthesia of the tongue and lip. Phentolamine is a non-selective α-adrenergic receptor antagonist. The blockade of $\alpha 1$-adrenergic receptors in smooth muscles of the blood vessels will result in vasodilatation, reversing the action of the vasoconstrictor. Therefore, injection of phentolamine would enhance the transport of the anaesthetic towards the blood circulation.

For use in the dental office, cartridges of 1.7 ml containing 0.4 mg phentolamine mesylate are available. They will be administered after the completion of the dental treatment. At the same location where the local anaesthetic has been injected, an equal volume (in ml) of the phentolamine mesylate is injected. The administration of phentolamine will reduce the time until the sensitivity of the soft tissue returns by 50–60 %.

3.3.8 Systemic Elimination

The aromatic part of the ester-type local anaesthetics is derived from para-amino benzoic acid (PABA). Ester anaesthetics are metabolised in the plasma by the enzyme pseudocholinesterase, which generates PABA analogues and amino alcohol. The PABA analogues are excreted in the urine mainly unaltered; the amino alcohol is further metabolised in the liver. Approximately 2 % of ester anaesthetics are excreted unchanged by the kidneys. The PABA analogues are responsible for the allergic reactions that frequently occur with the use of local anaesthetics of the ester type (▶ see Sect. 11.5).

Anaesthetics of the amide type are metabolised in the liver first by the cytochrome P_{450} system. This reaction is followed by conjugation, resulting in highly water-soluble metabolites that are excreted by the kidneys. Between 70 and 90 % of the amide anaesthetic is metabolised, and 10–30 % is excreted by the kidneys unchanged.

The velocity of degradation in the liver is reciprocally related to the toxicity. Prilocaine is metabolised fastest and consequently the least toxic amide-type local anaesthetic. Patients with severe liver insufficiency degrade amide-type local anaesthetics at a delayed rate, which increases the risk of a toxic effect (▶ see Sect. 12.6).

3.4   Additives to Local Anaesthetics

In addition to hydrochloric acid, to make the base form of local anaesthetic water soluble, several other ingredients are added to the solutions of local anaesthetics. The most important additives are vasoconstrictors and preservatives.

3.4.1 Vasoconstrictors

Vasoconstrictors are extremely important in the clinical use of local anaesthetics. Without these compounds, the clinical use of local anaesthetics in dentistry would be hampered by their limited duration of action, as most anaesthetics produce vasodilatation. Exceptions are mepivacaine and prilocaine. Vasoconstrictors reduce the blood flow at the site of injection, which reduces the spread and resorption of the local anaesthetic, thereby enhancing the duration and intensity. In addition, vasoconstriction delays the absorption, which decreases systemic toxicity. Therefore, the vasoconstrictors adrenaline (also known as epinephrine) and felypressin are added to the local anaesthetics used in dentistry.

Adrenaline is an endogenous compound, released into the blood by the adrenal medulla, with a half-life of only a few minutes. Nervous or anxious people may have increased blood levels of adrenaline from fear of dental treatment. Vasoconstriction by adrenaline is achieved by stimulation of α_1-adrenergic receptors of the smooth muscles of the vessel wall. The maximum dose of adrenaline for adults is 200 µg.

Felypressin (octapressin) is a synthetic vasoconstrictor, derived from vasopressin (antidiuretic hormone). The vasoconstrictive activity of felypressin mainly originates from inducing constriction of the venous part of the circulation. This might be important for the treatment of post-operative bleeding. An epinephrine-containing anaesthetic will mask a post-operative bleeding, while anaesthetics with felypressin will not. The duration of action of felypressin is also longer than that of adrenaline. For adults, the maximum dose of felypressin is 5.4 μg.

The use of vasoconstrictors can have negative effects, both locally and systemically. The reduced blood flow decreases the pH of the tissue, which shifts the equilibrium reaction towards the ionised form of the anaesthetic. This reduces the penetration of the local anaesthetic in the nerve and diminishes the anaesthetic effect. In addition, decreased blood flow may have a negative effect on wound healing. A third local disadvantage is that a 'rebound' effect may occur as soon as the vasoconstrictor has worn off, due to the accumulation of degradation products; because of increased blood flow, there is an increased risk of secondary haemorrhage. After intravasal injection of an adrenaline-containing local anaesthetic, blood pressure and heart frequency will increase. In healthy patients, however, this does not necessarily result in an emergency.

3.4.2 Preservatives

Methyl- and propylparaben are antibacterial agents (1 mg/ml). Because of their chemical structure, closely related to PABA, they frequently induce allergic reactions. Therefore, these preservatives are currently hardly ever added to local anaesthetic solutions.

Another preservative is bisulphite (0.3–2.0 mg/ml). This antioxidant is necessary to prevent oxidation of the vasoconstrictor potentially present, usually adrenaline. However, not only does bisulphite decrease the pH of the solution, but also some individuals may develop an allergy to this antioxidant.

3.4.3 Additives to Topical Anaesthetics

In the case of topical anaesthesia, a relatively highly concentrated solution of local anaesthetic is applied to the mucosa. The anaesthetic penetrates the surface tissue, and the subsequent resorption can occur very rapidly. Topical anaesthesia is therefore characterised by the rapid onset (2 min) and short length (10 min) of anaesthesia. For dental practice, topical anaesthetics are available as spray, gel and ointment. Disadvantages of the lidocaine-containing, alcohol-based spray are the rapid spread of the fluid over the mucosa and the unpleasant taste. To reduce the unpleasant taste, flavouring substances such as banana essence, menthol and saccharin are added. In addition, polyethylene glycol is incorporated as a modifying agent. Direct administration of the spray to the mucosa shows a very high degree of absorption. For example, ten puffs of a lidocaine spray 10 % are almost equivalent to an intravenous injection of 100 mg. Another disadvantage of using a spray is that it causes irritation of the mucosa, especially in the oropharynx, probably induced by parabens added to sprays as preservatives.

In the gel form, lidocaine is present as chloride, with methyl- and propyl-hydroxybenzoate as preservatives. To enhance the adhesion to the mucosa, hypromellose is used as an additive. In addition, several flavours can be added to the gel. By application of a gel at the injection site, the dose of topical anaesthetic can be kept very low and local. Sometimes patients with aphthous ulcers apply lidocaine gel before eating, enabling them to eat normally.

In ointments, lidocaine is present as base, with polyethylene and propylene glycol added as modifying agents. The ointment contains, like the anaesthetic gel, cellulose derivatives to improve the attachment to the oral mucosa. No further additives are present, but the possibility exists to add essences to improve the taste. Such essences are available in supermarkets, improve the taste and offer a choice for the (young) patient. Only a limited amount of lidocaine ointment 5 % is necessary to achieve an anaesthetic effect.

General Practical Aspects

J.A. Baart

© Springer International Publishing Switzerland 2017
J.A. Baart, H.S. Brand (eds.), *Local Anaesthesia in Dentistry*, DOI 10.1007/978-3-319-43705-7_4

4

In dentistry, local anaesthesia is often necessary in order to be able to treat patients. Local anaesthesia facilitates a painless treatment, so that the patient's comfort is maximal during the treatment and so that the dentist is able to work calmly, with concentration and precision. This benefits the end result and the way this is achieved. Local anaesthesia is also used for diagnostic purposes to identify the cause of pain in the face, using selective anaesthesia. It is also used to prevent short- or long-term postoperative pain.

4.1   Use of Local Anaesthetics

Local anaesthesia may be applied preventatively when the dentist expects that dental treatment will be uncomfortable or painful and/or if the patient cannot bear pain very well. In other cases, the anaesthetic is only used once pain does actually occur and/or if the patient indicates that he/she is no longer able to bear the pain.

Depending on the experience of the dentist and his/her knowledge of the patient's character, there is usually a preference for using preventative anaesthesia. This helps to increase the patient's confidence in the dentist and the treatment ('rather proactive than reactive'). Of course it makes a difference whether local anaesthesia is used for a sub- or supragingival cleaning, a cavity preparation, a crown or operative removal of a wisdom tooth or an extensive periodontal 'flap' procedure. There is also a difference in the way local anaesthetics are used for adults and children (▶ see Chap. 9). ◘ Table 4.1 provides some general guidelines for the use of various techniques and indications for local anaesthesia (◘ Box 4.1).

4.2   Indications and Contraindications

Before administration of an anaesthetic, the dentist must first explain why it is necessary. Indications and contraindications only have reference to the individual patient. Therefore, careful consideration must be made in the case of each patient, whether or not it is possible or suitable to use anaesthesia. This involves obtaining a good medical history and making enquiries related to previous experiences with local anaesthesia. The medical history should be well structured, systematic and preferably made in written form. Negative findings such as 'no medication', 'no allergies' and 'no bleeding tendency' must also be documented. When enquiring about earlier experiences, it is important to continue asking for details, e.g. what the patient means by 'collapse' and 'allergy to adrenaline'. Some physical reactions may be based on a nervous, mostly involuntary response. Examples of these are dizziness, nausea, stomach pains, fainting and sweating.

☐ **Table 4.1** General guidelines and indications for the use of various techniques to administer local anaesthesia

Therapeutic/diagnostic	Lower jaw	Upper jaw
Cleaning		
Limited	INF	INF
Extensive	MB	INF
Filling/crown	MB + INF	INF
Endodontics	MB (IL)	INF
Extraction	MB + INF	INF
Periodontal surgery	MB + INF	HTA, INA, PN
M$_3$ inferior/superior extraction	MB + INF	HTA, INF
Implantation	MB + INF	HTA + PN
Pre-implantological surgery	MB + MNB	HTA + PN
Central of peripheral pain?	MB	HTA + PN + INF
Dentogenic or non-dentogenic?	MB	INA, HTA
Which tooth?	IL	IL or INF

HTA = high tuberosity anaesthesia (block anaesthesia); IL = intraligamental nerve anaesthesia; INA = infraorbital nerve anaesthesia; INF = infiltration anaesthesia; MB = mandibular block (block anaesthesia); MNB = mental nerve block; NNP = nasopalatine nerve anaesthesia; PN = (greater) palatine nerve block

Box 4.1 Anaesthesia During Dental Hygiene Treatment
Whether anaesthesia is necessary during scaling and root planing should be decided jointly by the dentist and patient. The patient knows his sensitivity to pain from previous experiences. The dentist knows whether supra- or subgingival scaling has to be performed, the depth of the pockets, the severity of the furcation defect and the extent of the periodontal inflammation. A local anaesthetic not only serves the comfort of the patient but also improves the quality of the dental hygiene treatment. An anaesthetised patient will lie more relaxed in the dental chair, the vasoconstrictor will reduce bleeding of the periodontium, and the dentist is able to work calmly. Therefore, the question is whether infiltration anaesthesia, block anaesthesia or a combination of both should be applied.

If only the periodontium has to be anaesthetised, infiltration anaesthesia will suffice. The vasoconstrictor will work optimally. A disadvantage of infiltration anaesthesia is that the anaesthetic effect disappears rather rapidly, which makes repeated injections necessary. The pulp is not anaesthetised, a major disadvantage in people with sensitive teeth.

Regional block anaesthesia, on the other hand, will anaesthetise a larger area than necessary. The lower lip and tongue will also be anaesthetised, increasing the risk of postoperative automutilation. With block anaesthesia, the vasoconstrictor will not reduce the bleeding of the periodontium. In practice, therefore, a combination of infiltration and block anaesthesia is preferred for more extensive treatment.

4

Other symptoms, however, may indicate an overdose, allergic reactions or interaction with the prescribed medication that the patient is already taking. ◘ Table 12.1 gives recommendations for the use of local anaesthetics in medically compromised patients.

After explaining the nature of the anaesthesia, the dentist must verify whether the patient has understood this explanation. The patient may have additional questions that have to be answered first. Eventually the dentist will ask, more or less explicitly, for permission to anaesthetise (informed consent). If a patient does not protest against the use of a local anaesthetic, this does not mean that he/she is giving implicit permission (▶ see Chap. 13)!

4.3   Instruments

For the application of local anaesthetics in dentistry, almost exclusively use is made of glass cartridges with anaesthetic fluid, disposable needles and an aspirating syringe that can be sterilised. As an alternative, disposable aspirating syringes can be used.

4.3.1 Cartridges

The glass cartridges usually contain 1.7–1.8 ml of anaesthetic fluid, although in the UK also 2.2 ml cartridges are available. In this textbook, recommendations are based on cartridges of 1.8 ml. The cartridge is closed, on one side by a synthetic diaphragm and on the other side by a synthetic stopper that may or may not be prepared for aspiration (◘ Fig. 4.1). The outside of the cartridge is printed with the name, composition and vasoconstrictor of the local anaesthetic. This information is printed onto the glass or on a thin plastic foil. The latter ensures that, if the glass breaks (with intraligamental anaesthesia), the fragments are held together by the plastic foil and do not end up in the oral cavity (◘ Fig. 4.2).

Cartridges are delivered in sterile packing, and on the cartridges the expiry date, the stock number and other information are written (◘ Fig. 4.3). A cartridge that has just been unpacked does not need to be disinfected before use with, for example, chlorhexidine in alcohol. It is also not advisable, for various reasons, to preserve cartridges in disinfectant fluid.

The packs of cartridges can be kept at room temperature or in the fridge. If kept in a fridge, they must be taken out in plenty of time before use and have reached room temperature. Having a cold anaesthetic fluid injected is particularly painful.

Fig. 4.1 **a** Top of an anaesthetic cartridge with synthetic diaphragm, into which the needle can be pierced. **b, c** Bottom of an anaesthetic cartridge with synthetic stopper that is **b** or is not **c** prepared for aspiration

Fig. 4.2 **a, b** Glass anaesthetic cartridges with plastic foil on which the composition of the contents are noted; articaine 4 % with adrenaline 1:100.000 **a** and prilocaine 3 % with octapressin **b**

4

Fig. 4.3 Cartridges are delivered in a sterile packing and are printed with the stock number and use by date

4.3.2 **Needles**

All needles used for local anaesthesia in dentistry are disposable and meant for single use only. The length of the needle is given in millimetres. A long needle is approx. 35 mm, a short one is approx. 25 mm, and an extra-short needle is approx. 12 mm. These needles are suitable for regional anaesthesia, infiltration anaesthesia and intraligamental anaesthesia, respectively (■ Fig. 4.4a). The diameter of the needle is measured in terms of gauge. The smaller the gauge number, the larger the needle's diameter. Most needles used in dentistry have a gauge of 25–30. A number higher than 30 (i.e. very thin) should not be used, because aspiration of blood is then no longer possible. It is a misunderstanding that thinner needles are less painful than wider ones. Needles are made of surgical steel. The outside must be polished, and the 'bevel' should be carefully grinded without burrs. Therefore, it is primarily the needle pressure, the outflow speed of the liquid, the temperature and the pH that determine how painful an injection is. Reducing the needle diameter means that, with equal pressure, the liquid will be injected faster. Currently, so-called thin wall needles are in use, which have a wider lumen than the conventional needle.

The needle is contained in a metal or plastic cover. Part of the needle sticks out at the bottom and is meant to be inserted through the synthetic diaphragm into the anaesthetic fluid. The other part of the needle is used to actually apply the injection. The needles are packed in sterile packing and have two plastic caps that are removed from the needle by unscrewing and simultaneously bending them slightly (■ Fig. 4.4b). After use the needle should be preferably completely disassembled and disposed of in a sharps container. The cap should not be placed back over the needle. Recapping is incorrect dentistry.

◘ Fig. 4.4 **a** Different types of injection needles for local anaesthesia. From top to bottom: intraligamental needle, short needle for infiltration anaesthesia, longer needle for block anaesthesia (e.g. for the mandibular block) and a 'thin wall needle' for block anaesthesia. **b** Removal of the back of the disposable needle with a turning and bending motion. **c** After use, the disposable needle is unscrewed using the upper side of a 'sharps' container

The needle is particularly flexible and can bend easily during mandibular anaesthesia. This does not, however, cause the needle to break. Sometimes it is necessary to bend the needle a little before injecting. This is the case with, for example, anaesthesia in the floor of the mouth, in the palatine canal and with high-tuberosity anaesthesia. Even here the needle will not break. Repetitive bending of the needle may, however, lead to breakage, which is a serious complication (▶ see Sect. 10.1).

4.3.3 The Syringe

The syringe can usually be sterilised and is therefore made of rustproof steel. Chromed steel is not advisable. Some cartridge syringes are made of plastic and thus disposable. There are two different types of syringes: an insert type and a snap-in type (see ◘ Fig. 4.5). In addition to standard-size syringes, there are also syringes available for smaller hands (◘ Fig. 4.5d).

The front of the cartridge syringe has screw thread into which the mantle of the needle can be screwed. The back of the syringe has a ring to facilitate manual aspiration. The syringe plunger must be linked to the synthetic stopper of the glass cartridge with

◘ Fig. 4.5   a Syringes of rustproof steel, insert type (*above*) and snap-in type (*below*). **b** Insert-type syringe – by pulling back the plunger, the cartridge is laid into place in the syringe. **c** Snap-in type syringe – the cartridge is placed in the syringe; once the plunger is slightly pulled back, the syringe is snapped open. **d** Standard-size cartridge syringe and one for smaller hands (*below*)

anaesthetic fluid. This can be done in a variety of ways. Sometimes there is a little harpoon or spiral corkscrew that pierces the synthetic stopper. Other possibilities are a little cap or a blunt offset bulb that fits into a prepared opening at the back of the cartridge's synthetic stopper (see ◘ Fig. 4.6).

Both the insert- and snap-in-type syringes have a spring mechanism that aids automatic aspiration. By decreasing the pressure on the plunger, a few microlitres are sucked into the syringe, so it is easy to see whether the point of the needle is intravasal (◘ Fig. 4.7).

To prepare the cartridge syringe, the following steps are taken. First, a cartridge is placed in the syringe by pulling the plunger back slightly (insert type) or snapping it into the syringe (snap-in type). Then the plunger with harpoon, corkscrew, cap or bulb is pressed into the back of the synthetic stopper to enable aspiration. After this, the mantle of the needle is screwed onto the screw thread of the front of the syringe. By applying light pressure, one can now verify whether the syringe is ready to be used.

Once the first cartridge of anaesthetic fluid has been injected, it is possible that another cartridge will need to be applied, for example, in another part of the patient's mouth. The plunger is disconnected from the back of the synthetic stopper and pulled back completely.

■ **Fig. 4.6**   Syringes for manual aspiration, with either a corkscrew (*left*) at the end of the plunger or a little cap (*right*)

■ **Fig. 4.7**   Syringe used for aspirating with a visible trace of blood in the cartridge

The cartridge can then be taken out and replaced by a new one. Once this is done, the plunger with harpoon, corkscrew, cap or bulb is carefully reinserted into the back of the synthetic stopper. This must be done *before* the syringe is checked for use because otherwise anaesthetic fluid will have leaked out of the needle already.

If during aspiration a considerable amount of blood appears in the anaesthetic fluid, the cartridge must be replaced to ensure that when aspirating again there is no risk of the injection being given intravasally.

A combination of needle, cartridge and syringe is reserved for one patient only. In order to avoid confusion, this combination must, therefore, be prepared per patient and not in advance.

Relatively new are so-called auto-aspirating syringes. Aspiration occurs when the small 'chimney' on the front of the syringe is pushed against the plastic membrane of the carpule (◘ Figs. 4.8).

When the needle point is at the target site and one prepares to inject, the cartridge is moved forwards 2 mm over the membrane. When the pressure on the content of the cartridge is interrupted, the cartridge will rebound due to the elasticity of the membrane, and aspiration will take place.

Several types of disposable syringes are available, with a fixed extra-short, short or long needle. Only the cartridge with the chosen anaesthetic has to be added. After the injection, a covering shield is moved over the needle. This shield can no longer be moved backwards, which eliminates the risk of needle stick injuries (◘ Fig. 4.9 and Box 4.2).

◘ **Fig. 4.8** Detail of the inner side of an auto-aspiration syringe

◘ **Fig. 4.9** Assembly of a disposable syringe with a short needle. A cartridge is placed in the syringe **a**. The handle is snapped on the syringe **b**. After removal of the 'cap', the syringe is ready for use **c**. After use, the shield is moved forwards (do not 'recap') **d**. The shield snaps tight and can no longer be moved backwards **e**. Disassembly **f**

◘ **Fig. 4.9** continued

> **Box 4.2   Considerations for Choosing Disposable Syringes**
> Sterilisable cartridge syringes have a long life. Auto-aspirating types of
> sterilisable syringes comply with all current safety regulations. Why
> should one use disposable syringes when one already possesses
> sterilisable cartridge syringes?
> - Cost considerations: The cleaning and sterilising of sterilisable
>   cartridge syringes are more costly than one realises,
>   considering salary of staff and energy costs.
> - Environmental considerations: Cleaning and autoclaving are
>   harmful to the environment. Disposable syringes are
>   frequently manufactured of recycled or degradable plastic.
> - Safety considerations: Needle stick injuries are extremely
>   annoying for members of the dental team. If a dentist pricks
>   himself/herself, it is usually with a needle that has not been
>   used yet. If a dental assistant pricks himself/herself, it is usually
>   with a used needle. Disposable syringes reduce the risk of
>   needle stick injuries.
> - Practical considerations: (Automatic) aspiration as well as
>   changing a cartridge is more easy in a sterilisable cartridge
>   syringe than in a disposable one.
> - Patient considerations: It can be expected that patients will
>   more and more frequently ask questions about the safety and
>   sterility of an injection. Your sterilisable syringes are, without
>   doubt, well cleaned and sterilised. However, with a disposable
>   syringe, one can point out to the patient that the syringe has
>   been obtained directly from the manufacturer and has never
>   been used by someone else.

4

Fig. 4.10   a, b Intraligamental syringe; disassembled **a** and assembled **b**. Light pressure on the handle enables a strong and uniform outflow of the anaesthetic fluid. The metal cover protects the glass cartridge from breakage

Syringes for intraligamental anaesthesia have a deviant form. Intraligamental anaesthesia requires high pressure, which increases the risk of breaking the glass cartridge. ▪ Fig. 4.10 shows an example of a sterilisable intraligamental syringe. The plunger is moved forwards with a pumping motion. The cartridge is protected against breakage or its consequences, as it is completely surrounded by metal. In order to prevent ischaemic damage to the periodontal ligament as a result of the fluid pressure and/or vasoconstrictor, it is advisable to wait briefly between each pumping motion. Intraligamental anaesthesia applied with a microprocessor-controlled pump (the Wand®) does not have this problem, since the outflow speed is very low (▸ see Chap. 9). In addition to sterilisable syringes for intraligamental anaesthesia, there is also a disposable version available. This syringe has the advantage that the pumping mechanism raises very slowly. As a result, the pressure in the tissue is so low that the injection is not sensed by the patient (▪ Fig. 4.11).

Fig. 4.11   Disposable syringe for intraligamental anaesthesia. The red handle comes up gradually

Fig. 4.12 **a** Topical anaesthesia with use of lidocaine spray 10 %. Application is done with a roll of cotton wool or a cotton bud. **b** Topical anaesthesia with use of lidocaine gel 5 %. Two different flavours: mint and cherry aroma

4.4   **Topical Anaesthesia**

Occasionally it is advisable to apply preliminary anaesthesia. The benefits lie partly in the anaesthesia of the point of injection and partly in psychological factors. Preliminary anaesthesia for intraligamental and block anaesthesia has a limited effect and is therefore not advocated. Preliminary anaesthesia may be beneficial for infiltration anaesthesia. Topical anaesthesia is available as spray and gel (Fig. 4.12). The gel is preferred, as it has better adhesion to the oral mucosa and is available with various flavours (mint, cherry). If a patient can choose, this will increase the informed consent during the subsequent injection.

In contrast to what is stated in the accompanying guidelines, it is better not to use anaesthetic spray directly in the mouth. Lidocaine spray 10 % is very easily absorbed by the mucosa of the oral-throat cavity, which increases the risk of children being overdosed. Moreover, the spray nozzle must be cleaned and sterilised again, even after a single use. It is therefore better to apply the spray fluid or anaesthetic gel to a roll of cotton wool or the tip of a cotton bud. This allows the dentist, the dental assistant or patients themselves to apply a very precise preliminary anaesthesia. It is enough to apply the spray fluid or gel 2–3 minutes before inserting the injection needle (Box 4.3).

> **Box 4.3**
> In dental treatment, it is not enough to simply apply topical anaesthesia without following up with infiltration or regional block anaesthesia, since the depth and duration of surface anaesthesia are limited.

4.5   Position of the Patient and Dentist

In dentistry, local anaesthetics are often applied preventatively, i.e. before any pain occurs due to the treatment. Some dentists therefore anaesthetise patients while they are sitting up in the dentist's chair. This is not right. The view into the mouth is not optimal, the position of the lamp is not ideal, and, in case of a vasovagal collapse (▶ Sect. 11.2), the patient may fall off the chair forwards. It is therefore sensible to apply local anaesthesia with the dentist and patient in the position they have during the subsequent treatment. This means that usually the patient is anaesthetised in a semi-horizontal to horizontal position. A right-handed dentist sits next to the dental chair in a 9–1 o'clock position, while the assistant sits in a 2–3 o'clock position.

During administration of the anaesthetic, the dentist should hold the patient's head steady with the arm and free non-injecting hand (◘ Fig. 4.13). Any unexpected movement of the patient will then not lead to any self-injury or injection in the wrong place. Moreover, especially with mandibular block anaesthesia and infraorbital nerve anaesthesia, it is easier to find the point of injection with the steadying and feeling hand. The possibility of the dentist pricking his/her own hand if the patient's head moves unexpectedly is very slight and not unduly dangerous for the dentist's health if it happens with an unused needle. Nevertheless, some dentists have a dental mirror or wooden spatula in the non-injecting hand to protect themselves from self-injection.

Just before the needle actually penetrates the mucosa, the mucosa is stretched, and the dentist carefully pinches the patient's

◘ **Fig. 4.13**   The dentist holds the head of the patient steady with the free gloved hand

lip or cheek to mask the prick. An intravasal injection is avoided by aspirating before injecting and repeating this after every change of position of the needle. The injection itself must be given very slowly. The injection speed may be a little higher for free mucosa. The dentist must continually ask for the patient's experience of the local anaesthesia both during and directly after the injection. Young and nervous patients should be given compliments for the way they handled the anaesthesia.

It is not correct to anaesthetise the patient and then ask him/her to sit in the waiting room until the anaesthesia has taken effect. Local anaesthesia takes effect in between 30 and 180 seconds, and this does not justify leaving a recently anaesthetised patient in the waiting room without proper supervision. During or immediately after an injection, unexpected reactions may occur.

If the patient has an undesired reaction during or after applying a local anaesthetic, the dentist must react calmly. It is important that the dentist gives a good explanation and, if necessary, an apology. For example, a patient could experience palpitations after an intravascular injection with a local anaesthetic containing adrenaline. 'Blanching' may appear in the face. In this case a comforting explanation will suffice. If a nerve is pricked, e.g. the inferior alveolar nerve, lingual nerve or mental nerve, the patient will need more than an explanation and calming word. In this case, the feeling may be altered for days, weeks and sometimes months (▶ see Chap. 10).

Undesired reactions to local anaesthesia may, of course, also be related to the dentist's skill and method of injection. Assembling the anaesthetic syringe in front of the patient and checking whether the anaesthetic fluid is ready by ostentatiously tapping the syringe and holding it to the ceiling to release any air bubbles do not reassure the average patient. A sudden or rough application of a local anaesthetic must be avoided. The injection must be given extremely slowly anywhere in the mouth and especially in the palatal mucosa.

4.6 Verification of Effectiveness

To verify the effectiveness of the anaesthesia, the dentist should first ask the patient open questions: 'Do you already notice any change yet? What do you feel? Could you indicate where it is tingling or where it feels numb?' If the patient's answers are unclear, the dentist can help the patient by asking: 'What about the lip? And the tongue?' If necessary, he/she can ask about differences in feeling: 'Does it have the same feeling as this side? If I touch here, does it feel the same as there?' The dentist must avoid asking closed questions that can be answered with a 'yes' because the answers are unreliable. 'Is the lip tingling already? And the tongue?' must not be asked after anaesthesia. Some combinations of anaesthesia may lead to incorrect information from the patient on the effects of the local anaesthesia. If mandibular block anaesthesia is directly followed by infiltration anaesthesia in the premolar area, a one-sided numbed lower lip does not say much. Therefore, it is better in these cases to first give the mandibular block, to wait for a more or less spontaneous reaction from the patient, who may say the lower lip has begun to tingle, and only then to continue with infiltration anaesthesia buccal to the lower premolars.

It is proper practice towards the patient to give a little prick with, for example, a dental probe in order to test the anaesthesia before proceeding to the painful treatment. An ineffective anaesthesia that is not noticed by the dentist, followed by a painful treatment, damages the patient's confidence in the dentist and his/her treatment. In certain cases, the dentist may use additional techniques such as suggestive relaxation, hypnosis and inhalation sedatives. Some patients may also be given medication that relaxes or makes them drowsy, or general anaesthesia, which is usually given intravenously (◻ Box 4.4).

> **Box 4.4   Afterpain**
> After dental treatment, afterpain may occur. This is not caused by the administration of local anaesthesia but by tissue damage during dental treatment. Depending on the dental treatment, the expected afterpain may be severe or limited. In the latter case, the dentist can advise: 'If afterpain develops, you can take a 500 milligram tablet of paracetamol (acetaminophen), not more than five per day'. However, when severe afterpain is expected, based on the extensiveness of the dental treatment, the dentist will prescribe an analgesic, e.g. an NSAID. When an NSAID is prescribed, possible contraindications and the potential concomitant prescription of a stomach protector should be taken into account.

4.7   Teaching Anaesthesia Techniques

The regular curriculum of dental schools usually comprises most infiltration and regional block anaesthetic techniques. Additional techniques can be learned during postgraduate courses.

Several studies have shown that training of injection techniques on an anaesthesia model before the first injection in a patient has added value (◻ Fig. 4.14). To learn injection techniques with such

🔲 **Fig. 4.14** A modern, interactive model to train several injection techniques (Courtesy of DRSK Development AB, Sweden)

a model correctly, several requirements have to be considered with regard to the implementation in the anaesthesia course:

– Practicing of students on the model should be supervised one on one by an experienced staff member.
– The training model should resemble reality closely. This means that soft tissues, such as lips, cheeks and buccal sulcus, should be present.
– There should be direct feedback of correct anaesthesia with light and/or sound signals. Preferably, the training model should differentiate whether the needle is inserted correctly, almost correctly or incorrectly.
– The training model should also be suitable for additional techniques, such as high-tuberosity anaesthesia (▶ Sect. 7.1.1), infraorbital nerve block (▶ Sect. 7.2), Gow-Gates technique (▶ Sect. 7.5.1) and the Vazirani-Akinosi method (▶ Sect. 7.5.2).

Local Anaesthesia in the Upper Jaw

J.A. Baart

© Springer International Publishing Switzerland 2017
J.A. Baart, H.S. Brand (eds.), *Local Anaesthesia in Dentistry*, DOI 10.1007/978-3-319-43705-7_5

5.1   Introduction

The sensory innervation of the upper jaw arises from the second trunk of the trigeminal nerve, the maxillary nerve. This main branch of the trigeminal nerve leaves the neurocranium via the foramen rotundum, reaches the pterygopalatine fossa and runs straight through as the infraorbital nerve, branching off many times along its course. With regard to local anaesthesia in the upper jaw, the following branches are of importance:

- The greater and lesser palatine nerves
- The posterior, middle and anterior superior alveolar nerves
- The infraorbital nerve (■ Fig. 5.1)

Thus, the main trunk of the maxillary nerve can be reached via the greater palatine foramen, via the infraorbital foramen as well as from high behind the maxillary tuberosity. In practice, high-tuberosity anaesthesia is the only practical regional block anaesthesia for almost the entire maxillary nerve. Therefore,

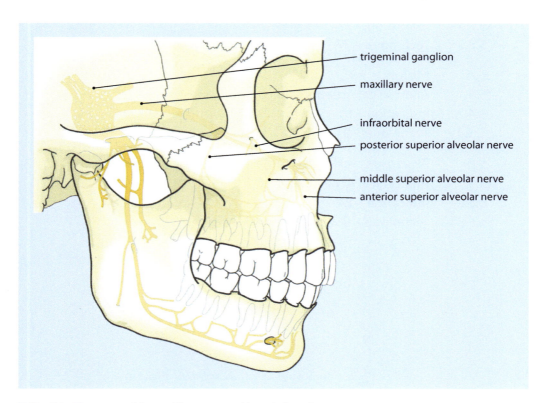

■ **Fig. 5.1**   The course of the maxillary nerve and its main branches

this regional block anaesthesia technique is used for surgical procedures.

For dental procedures in the upper jaw, infiltration anaesthesia is commonly used. The cortical bone of the outer surface of the upper jaw is relatively thin, which facilitates the diffusion of local anaesthetic fluid. All (buccal) roots of the upper teeth can be reached in this way. The palatine roots of the molars and possibly the premolars are anaesthetised by infiltration anaesthesia of the branches of the greater palatine nerve and those of the nasopalatine nerve. Regional block anaesthesia is also possible via the greater palatine foramen and the nasopalatine canal.

Infiltration anaesthesia of the upper jaw is particularly effective, unless an injection is made into an inflamed area. Regional block anaesthesia of the greater palatine, nasopalatine and infraorbital nerves is equally effective. In cases of regional block anaesthesia using a high-tuberosity block, it is usually only the posterior superior alveolar and medial branches that are numbed but sometimes also the palatine and infraorbital nerves.

5.2 Incisors and Canines

5.2.1 Anatomical Aspects

Before leaving the infraorbital foramen, the infraorbital nerve branches off in the infraorbital canal towards the incisors and canines, the anterior superior alveolar nerves. These nerve branches provide the sensory innervation of the incisor and canine pulp, as well as the vestibular fold, the gingiva, the periosteum and the bone. They anastomose with small branches of the other vestibular side (◘ Fig. 5.2). The nasopalatine nerve leaves the incisive foramen and provides the sensory innervation of the palatine bone, periosteum and mucosa (◘ Fig. 5.3). Because of the relatively thin and porous nature of the maxilla's cortical bone, an extraperiosteal (infiltration) anaesthetic can spread easily within the maxillary bone.

The apices of the root of the central incisor and canine are found on the buccal side of the bone, whilst the apex of the lateral incisor is found on the palatal side. This must be taken into consideration when infiltration anaesthetics are given, especially when used for an apicoectomy. The anterior superior alveolar branches run from high lateral to low medial. For this reason, infiltration anaesthetics may best be applied laterally, just above the apex.

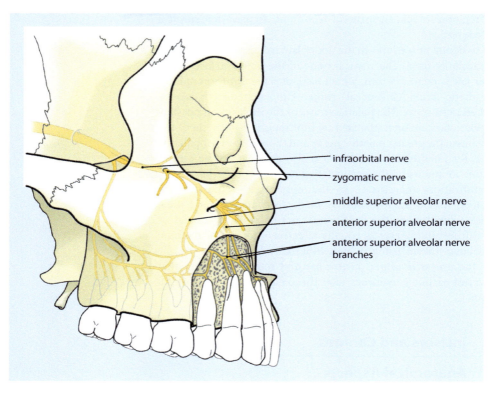

Fig. 5.2   Branches of the infraorbital nerve, before and after its exit via the infraorbital foramen

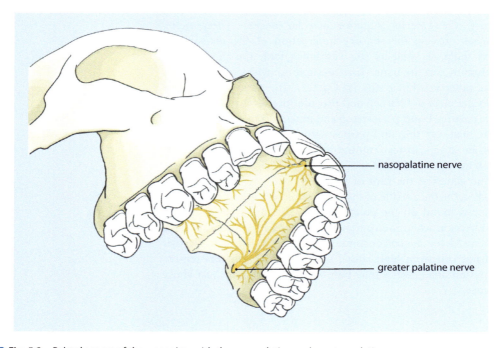

Fig. 5.3   Palatal aspect of the upper jaw with the nasopalatine and greater palatine nerves

5.2.2 **Indication**

For cavity preparations in the upper frontal teeth, buccal or labial infiltration anaesthesia is usually sufficient. The same applies to endodontic treatments. In cases where a cofferdam is used, or wedges, supplementary palatine anaesthesia is sometimes required. For crown preparations, it is sensible to use buccal and palatine infiltration anaesthesia.

For surgical procedures in the upper frontal teeth area, such as periodontal surgery, implants, extractions and apicoectomies, it is advisable to anaesthetise a larger area using regional block anaesthesia with supplementary infiltration anaesthesia. Because regional block anaesthesia is highly effective in this area, it can be directly followed by infiltration anaesthesia. The infraorbital and nasopalatine nerves can be reached via the infraorbital foramen and the nasopalatine canal. Infiltration anaesthesia is given in the buccal area and, if necessary, in the interdental (palatine) papillae. Nevertheless, there are exceptions where good anaesthesia is not achieved. The intraossal branches of the nasopalatine nerve are responsible for this. These smaller branches can be anaesthetised by an injection or the application of a cotton bud with anaesthetic ointment in the respective nostril (□ Fig. 5.4).

□ **Fig. 5.4** A cotton bud, soaked with a topical anaesthetic, in the nose of a patient in order to numb the intraossal branches of the nasopalatine nerve

5.2.3 **Technique**

Buccal infiltration anaesthesia of the upper frontal teeth is performed by lifting the lip with the free hand, gently pinching the lip and then piercing the mucosa of the buccal fold with the needle just above the apex of the respective tooth. The syringe is thereby held parallel to the longitudinal axis of the tooth. The needle is inserted no more than 3–5 mm, with the bevel directed towards the bone. Any contact of the needle point with the periosteum or the bone must be avoided, and the fluid must be injected slowly. Aspiration is recommended but not really necessary: there are no large blood vessels in this area (● Fig. 5.5).

Palatine infiltration anaesthesia is applied in the palatal gingiva of the respective tooth. This anaesthesia is particularly painful if the needle is moved up over the periosteum and when not injected extremely slowly. It is, therefore, sensible to insert the needle tangentially and not to move it up or to resort to palatine conduction anaesthesia for the central and lateral incisor (● Fig. 5.6a, b).

There is usually enough space for an anaesthetic around the canines at the transition between the vertical and horizontal sections of the palate. Here the space for injection fluid is maximum sub- and supraperiostally. Here too it is necessary to inject extremely slowly.

The required amount of local anaesthetic is small, both for buccal and palatine anaesthesia. For buccal anaesthesia, a

● **Fig. 5.5**   Infiltration anaesthesia for the I_1 superior right

■ **Fig. 5.6   a, b** Drawing **a** and photo **b** of regional block anaesthesia of the nasopalatine nerve. The needle is inserted at an angle into the incisive papilla to avoid damaging the nerve and bleeding from the vessels in the nasopalatine canal

quarter of a cartridge per tooth is sufficient, whereas a maximum of an eighth of a cartridge is needed for palatine anaesthesia. Sometimes it is necessary, in cases of periodontal or implant procedures, to inject anaesthetics into the interdental papillae, but this is painful for the patient. The dentist should, therefore, wait until the vestibular and/or palatine infiltration anaesthetic takes effect, before anaesthetising the interdental papillae.

▶ See Sect. 7.2 for a description of the block anaesthesia of the greater palatine and infraorbital nerves.

5.3   Premolars

5.3.1   Anatomical Aspects

Sensory innervation of the first and second premolars in the upper jaw arises from the superior alveolar nerve, via the middle and anterior superior alveolar branches. The middle superior alveolar branches run from high dorsal to low ventral, whereas the anterior superior alveolar branches come from the upper frontal area (■ Fig. 5.7).

Furthermore, because the lateral aspect of the upper jaw in this area is concave, the needle must be inserted a fraction from out to in, in order to inject close to the periosteum. The facial artery runs near the first premolar, high in the buccal fold, so aspiration prior to injection is indispensable.

The innervation of the premolar area arises on the palatal side from branches of the greater palatine nerve and also by smaller branches of the nasopalatine nerve that run dorsally (■ Fig. 5.3).

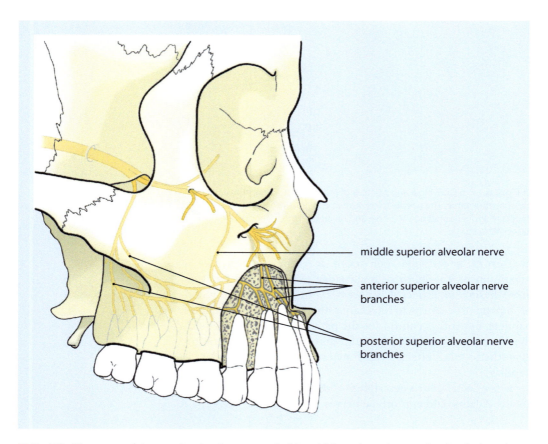

middle superior alveolar nerve

anterior superior alveolar nerve branches

posterior superior alveolar nerve branches

■ **Fig. 5.7**   The course of the superior alveolar nerve and of the middle and anterior superior alveolar branches

Besides the branches of the greater palatine nerve, the greater palatine artery and vein also run along the palatinal side, at the transition from vertical to horizontal aspect. An intravasal injection must be avoided by careful aspiration. Piercing the artery here also has the disadvantage of causing persistent bleeding from the needle hole. On the other hand, the injection must not be too superficial, since a high injective pressure is then required, which will result in a lot of pain, and ischemic necrosis of the palatal mucosa may occur after treatment (▶ see Sect. 10.8).

5.3.2 Indication

Buccal infiltration anaesthesia is sufficient for cavity preparations and endodontic treatments. If the first premolar of the upper jaw (P_{1sup}) has two diverging roots, additional palatal anaesthesia may be needed. This supplementary palatal anaesthesia is also needed for crown preparations. For surgical operations, such as periodontal surgery, implantology, extraction and apicoectomy, a larger anaesthetised area is required. For this reason, the anaesthetic is injected into the vestibular area at a point much higher than the apices, and in the palatinal area, the anaesthetic is injected near the apices at the point of transition from the horizontal to the vertical aspect. Though palatinal block anaesthesia is possible, it is discouraged as it requires two injections: one into the greater palatine foramen and another into the incisive papilla.

5.3.3 Technique

In the upper jaw, the transversal width of the alveolar process is narrowest in the area of the canines and rapidly increases in a dorsal direction. The apices of the roots of the first premolar lie, when they are bi-rooted and divergent, immediately below the buccal and palatal cortical bone, respectively. The single-rooted second premolar has an apex that lies more centrally in the alveolar process. This must be kept in mind when a local anaesthetic is applied here.

The corner of the patient's mouth is lifted, and the free hand should pinch the lip carefully, so that the needle's penetration into the buccal mucosa is hardly felt. With the point of the needle and the bevel directed towards the bone, a small amount of anaesthetic fluid is deposited just above and dorsal to the apex (◘ Fig. 5.8a, b). Aspiration for injection near the first premolar must be carried out in order to avoid an intravasal injection. If the fluid is injected intravasally, the patient will feel a short, sharp shot of pain in the

■ Fig. 5.8   a, b Drawing **a** and photo **b** of the infiltration anaesthesia of the P$_1$ superior right

face, and the skin of the cheek and lower eyelid will pale immediately (*blanching*) (▶ see Sect. 10.7).

The needle must be inserted from out to in. For restorative dental treatments, the needle point should be approx. 5 mm above the apex. For surgical procedures, more cranial infiltration anaesthesia is required. On the palatal side, the needle is inserted counter-laterally and vertically at the transition of the horizontal

◼ Fig. 5.9   Palatine infiltration anaesthesia of the P_1 and P_2 superior right. The needle is inserted from the left into the transitional area of the horizontal to vertical sections of the palate

---

Box 5.1   Selective Anaesthesia of the Upper Jaw
In the upper jaw, it is possible to anaesthetise teeth one by one. This can be used to locate the origin of pain, when it is not immediately clear which tooth is responsible for the complaints. This is especially the case with heavily restored teeth with (irreversible) pulpitis.

The procedure is as follows: You apply a very small amount of anaesthetic fluid on the buccal and, if necessary, on the palatal side near the apex of the tooth located ventral from the potential culprit. The patient will notice that the tooth becomes numb, but the pain will not disappear. This will avoid a placebo effect of your anaesthesia. Subsequently, you anaesthetise the tooth where you expect the pain to originate. After 2 min you ask whether the patient experiences the anaesthesia and how it is with the pain. When you have anaesthetised the tooth responsible for the pain effectively, the patient's relief will be expressed both verbally and non-verbally.

---

to the vertical aspect of the palate (◼ Fig. 5.9). After aspiration, the fluid is injected extremely slowly. The amount of anaesthetic fluid used in the buccal area is approx. 1 ml, and a maximum of 0.25 ml is used for the palatal side (◼ Box 5.1).

5.4   Molars

5.4.1   Anatomical Aspects

The posterior superior alveolar branches innervate the buccal side of the molar region of the upper jaw. These branches of the second

Fig. 5.10 The course of the superior alveolar nerve and the posterior superior alveolar branches

trunk of the trigeminal nerve originate high in the pterygopalatine fossa, and they run along the maxillary tuberosity to the low ventral area. They provide sensitivity in the M_3, M_2 and M_1 and the mucosa, gingiva, periosteum and bone (**Fig. 5.10**). The palatal mucosa and palatal root of the first molar in the upper jaw (M_{1sup}) are innervated by the greater palatine nerve, which also comes from the second trunk of the trigeminal nerve (see **Fig. 5.3**).

The zygomatic buttress is found in the buccal area above the apices of the M_{1sup}. The point of attachment can vary, however, so that an impermeable cortical layer of bone may sometimes be found lateral to the buccal roots of M_{1sup}, depending on the length of the vestibulary radices and the crest's point of attachment.

The position of the roots of the M_2 and the erupted M_{3sup} is more or less central in the bone, depending on the level of convergence. The transversal width of the alveolar process in the molar region is considerable, so that more anaesthetic fluid is needed for adequate numbing. The pterygoid venous plexus is found laterally high to the maxillary tuberosity.

5.4.2 Indication

For cavity preparations in the M_{1sup}, both buccal and palatal infiltration anaesthesia are required. For the second and third molar in the upper jaw, vestibulary anaesthesia will suffice for these indications. The same applies for endodental treatment of this area. If the M_{1sup} happens to have long buccal roots and/or a low-positioned zygomatic buttress, the infiltration anaesthesia must be applied behind the crest, i.e. higher and more dorsal.

For operative treatments such as periodontal surgery, implantology, extraction or apicoectomy (of the buccal roots), regional block anaesthesia is commonly used high above the maxillary tuberosity and at the position of the greater palatine foramen, supplemented with some buccal infiltration anaesthesia. The method of high-tuberosity anaesthesia is described in ► Sect. 7.1.1.

Regional block anaesthesia of the major palatine nerve is administered vertically from the counter-lateral corner of the mouth. The needle must not be inserted too deeply in the direction of the foramen in order to avoid damage to the nerve or piercing the artery. Aspiration prior to the actual injection is prescribed.

The amount of anaesthetic fluid for buccal infiltration anaesthesia should be approx. 1–1.5 ml. For palatine infiltration or block anaesthesia, no more than 0.25 ml is required.

Patients that are given an infiltration anaesthetic in the molar region of the upper jaw can have the impression that the anaesthetic has not worked. They compare the feeling they observe with the sensation that they know from an infiltration anaesthetic in the premolar region or the front teeth or from mandibular regional block anaesthesia. It is therefore wise to explain to patients this difference in sensation.

5.4.3 Technique

Infiltration anaesthesia on the buccal side of the upper molars is applied at an angle from the front. The jaw here is flat to convex. The zygomatic buttress sticks outwards and is found near the first molar. The point of the needle should be right above and dorsal to the apices (◘ Fig. 5.11a, b). For the first molar, it is occasionally necessary to inject behind the buttress and slightly higher, due to the inaccessibility of the buccal roots through the thick cortical bone. Sometimes branches of the posterior alveolar nerve run back

⬛ Fig. 5.11   a, b Drawing **a** and photo **b** of infiltration anaesthesia of the M_2 superior right. The needle is inserted slightly from out to in

to the area M_{1sup} in front of the buttress. For the palatal side, infiltration anaesthesia of the major palatine nerve at the first molar and regional block anaesthesia for the second and third molars are sufficient (⬛ Fig. 5.12a, b). For an extraction of the

◘ Fig. 5.12   a, b Drawing **a** and photo **b** of the palatal regional block anaesthesia of the greater palatine nerve. Careful aspiration prior to injection is required

second and erupted third molar, an injection of 0.25 ml fluid next to the gingival fold on the palatal side will suffice (◘ Fig. 5.13). ► See Sect. 7.1.1. for a description of the high-tuberosity anaesthesia method.

◘ **Fig. 5.13** Palatal infiltration anaesthesia of the gingiva on the level of the M_2 superior right

5.5   The Impacted Third Molar of the Upper Jaw

5.5.1 Anatomical Aspects

The impacted third molar of the upper jaw (M_{3sup}) is usually found completely in the maxillary tuberosity with a slight distovestibular inclination. Here, the buccal cortical bone is very thin. Slightly higher and in a more lateral position is the pterygoid venous plexus. The branches of the second trunk of the trigeminal nerve, and the maxillary artery and vein, run behind the tuberosity and higher in the pterygopalatine fossa. On the palatine side of the impacted M_{3sup} are the greater palatine foramen and the lesser palatine foramina, from which the palatine nerves branch off that innervate the palatine gingiva and the soft palate. The greater palatine arteries and vein also come from the greater palatine foramen. Therefore, the area lateral, dorsal and medial to the impacted M_{3sup} is richly innervated and vascularised. Here surgery outside of the periosteum is risky.

5.5.2 Indication

In the dental practice, local anaesthesia will only be used in this area for the removal of an impacted M_{3sup} or for harvesting bone for pre-implant treatment elsewhere in the mouth.

5.5.3 **Technique**

Anaesthesia of the entire greater palatine nerve and, if necessary, of the lesser palatine nerves is performed with regional block anaesthesia. The needle is brought forwards from the counter-lateral corner of the mouth in the direction of the greater and lesser palatine foramens (◘ Fig. 5.12a, b). Touching the nerve or piercing the artery must be avoided. For this reason, aspiration is necessary. Approximately 0.25 ml anaesthetic fluid is sufficient. Anaesthesia of the greater and lesser palatine nerves will induce numbness of a large part of the hard and soft palate. The patient may experience swallowing problems and a feeling of tightness. It is recommended to mention this risk in advance. Refer to ▶ Sect. 7.1.1 for information on the method of high-maxillary-tuberosity anaesthesia.

Local Anaesthesia in the Lower Jaw

J.A. Baart

© Springer International Publishing Switzerland 2017
J.A. Baart, H.S. Brand (eds.), *Local Anaesthesia in Dentistry*, DOI 10.1007/978-3-319-43705-7_6

6.1   Introduction

The buccal cortical bone at the premolars and molars of the lower jaw impedes the diffusion of anaesthetic fluid to the apices of these teeth or into the mandibular canal, located centrally in the jaw bone. Adults require mandibular block anaesthesia for an effective anaesthesia. In the area of the lower canines and incisors, the cortical bone is thinner, and the roots lie on the buccal side of the jaw. Here, infiltration anaesthesia is effective.

The mental nerve leaves the jaw through the mental foramen and innervates the buccal mucosa and gingiva, the lower lip and the skin of the chin. Therefore, anaesthetising the mental nerve will not anaesthetise the teeth in adults. However, in children the primary molars and permanent premolars are anaesthetised, because the apex of these teeth is reached through diffusion through the thinner and immature cortical bone.

The lingual side of the mandible is innervated by the lingual nerve. This nerve can be anaesthetised both by block anaesthesia and by infiltration anaesthesia. The dentist must avoid pricking the floor of the mouth too often as this increases the risk of a haematoma in combination with transport of bacteria with the injection needle. This may cause a phlegmonous infection of the mouth floor, a life-threatening complication.

Block anaesthesia of the buccal nerve is almost impossible. This nerve runs from high lingual and crosses the front side of the mandibular ramus above the occlusion plane. Then the buccal nerve continues caudo-ventrally to innervate the buccal mucosa and gingiva in the area of the (erupted) M_{3inf} to P_{2inf}. Because the height at which the buccal nerve crosses the mandibula varies, infiltration anaesthesia applied buccal to the respective teeth is a better technique to anaesthetise the gingiva and buccal mucosa (Figs. 6.1 and 6.2).

6.2   Incisors and Canines

6.2.1 Anatomical Aspects

Once the buccal and lingual nerves (and also the mylohyoid nerve) have separated from the trigeminal nerve, the nerve runs laterally and enters the mandibular foramen. The inferior alveolar nerve divides into a branch, the mental nerve, at the level of the mental foramen and then continues as the incisive nerve. The incisive nerve runs no longer in a bony canal and divides into little branches to the roots of the lower canines and incisors (Fig. 6.3). In the mandibular symphysis area, sensory anastomoses from the contralateral side are present, both lingually and buccally. This

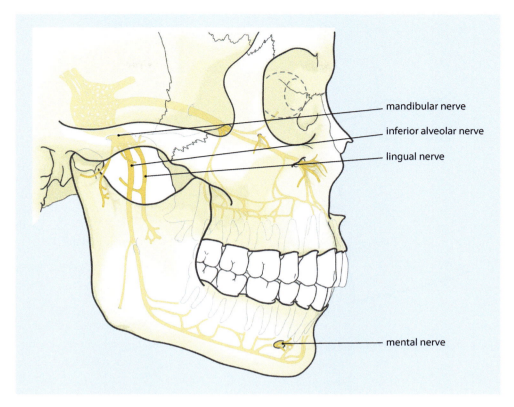

mandibular nerve

inferior alveolar nerve

lingual nerve

mental nerve

▣ Fig. 6.1 The path of the mandibular nerve with its main branches

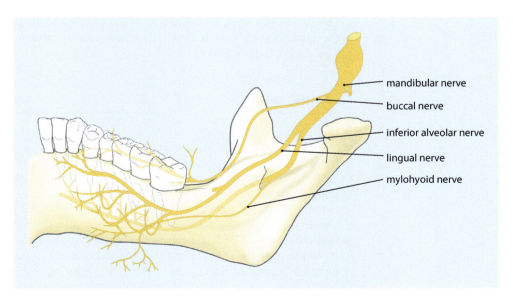

mandibular nerve

buccal nerve

inferior alveolar nerve

lingual nerve

mylohyoid nerve

▣ Fig. 6.2 Medial aspect of the path of the mandibular nerve and its branches: the buccal nerve, lingual nerve and inferior alveolar nerve

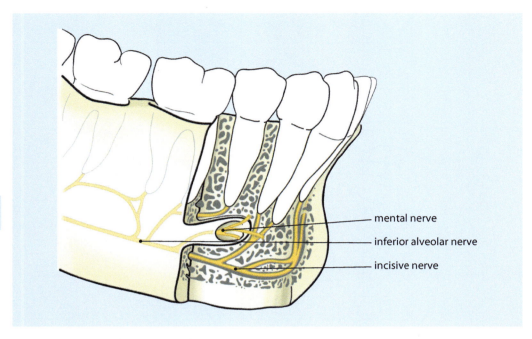

● **Fig. 6.3**   The path of the mental and incisive nerves

must be taken into account, particularly with extensive surgical treatment in the lower frontal area.

The roots of the lower incisors and canines are found against the buccal cortical bone. The mental muscle is attached to the jaw at the height of the I_{2inf} so that infiltration anaesthesia in this area can be painful and less effective.

6.2.2 **Indication**

Buccal infiltration anaesthesia will be sufficient for cavity preparations and endodontic treatment in the lower frontal area, unless a cofferdam and/or matrix bands and wedges are used. In that case, it is necessary to apply additional anaesthesia lingually, or perhaps in the interdental papilla on the lingual side.

Infiltration anaesthesia is also used for surgical treatment in the lower frontal area, in which case the needle is inserted more caudally to the apex. The dentist must take the sensory anastamoses into account by also anaesthetising the contralateral nerve branches. The point of attachment of the mimic muscles, such as the orbicularis oris muscle and the mental muscle, also requires special attention during anaesthesia. Injecting into these muscles causes bleeding, is painful and does not lead to a good anaesthesia of teeth.

Fig. 6.4 **a, b** Drawing **a** and photo **b** of infiltration anaesthesia of the I$_2$ inferior right. The buccal gingiva is also anaesthetised. In order to anaesthetise the lingual gingiva, it is necessary to inject into the floor of the mouth. **c** Lingual anaesthesia with a bent needle with the dentist in an 8–9 o'clock position. **d** Lingual anaesthesia with a non-bent needle with the dentist in an 11–1 o'clock position

6.2.3 **Technique**

For infiltration anaesthesia in the lower frontal area, the non-injecting hand pulls the lip forwards and pinches the lip softly at the moment the needle penetrates the mucosa. The needle is inserted right under the apex of the tooth that is to be anaesthetised, up to the bone with the bevel of the needle pointed to the bone. Preferably, the needle is inserted vertically and not pushed into the periosteum. The dentist sits or stands behind the patient in an 11–1 o'clock position. The same position is assumed for infiltration anaesthesia of the lingual mucosa and gingiva. When anaesthetising from an 8–9 o'clock position, it is better to bend the needle 45–90° for a lingual injection (■ Fig. 6.4). With lingual anaesthesia it is important to prevent a haematoma occurring. To anaesthetise the frontal teeth for periodontal reasons, a horizontal injection is advised: one at the left site and one at the right site of the frenulum.

Bilateral mandibular block anaesthesia, with additional local infiltration anaesthesia, is recommended for surgical treatment of the lower front, such as extensive pre-implantological treatments (e.g. a chin bone transplant) or implantological treatments (two or four dental implants). This reduces the required number of injections to a minimum, as well as the chance of haematomas and infections. Furthermore, a maximum of 4–6 ml of anaesthetic fluid will be sufficient.

In this situation it is recommended that the dentist administers the double-sided mandibular block first and then waits until the patient spontaneously indicates that the lower lip and border of the tongue have started to tingle. The dentist can then give a buccal infiltration anaesthesia and is convinced that the mandibular block 'works' well.

6.3   Premolars

6.3.1   Anatomical Aspects

Innervation of the premolars in the lower jaw takes place in the bone through the inferior alveolar nerve, buccal through the buccal nerve (at the P_{1inf} also through the mental nerve) and lingually through the lingual nerve. Because of the thickness and impermeability of the buccal cortical bone, infiltration anaesthesia is not reliable for the treatment of the (pulpa of) premolars in adult patients.

Use of block anaesthesia of the mandibular nerve, i.e. of the inferior alveolar and lingual nerves, is therefore a better choice, if necessary supplemented with local infiltration anaesthesia of the branches of the buccal nerve (◘ Fig. 6.5). The mental nerve is

◘ **Fig. 6.5** The path of the branches of the mandibular nerve in the premolar area

found lower than the apices, exactly between the two premolars. Block anaesthesia of the mental nerve branches must be given superficially to avoid damage of the mental nerve, with subsequent long-term anaesthesia of the lower lip half.

If a combination of block anaesthesia of the mandibular nerve and local infiltration is chosen, then the mandibular block must, of course, be given first. A supplementary infiltration anaesthetic is applied locally once the patient spontaneously reports that the lower lip half and edge of the tongue have begun to tingle. When the inferior alveolar nerve appears to be anaesthetised after block anaesthesia of the mandibular nerve, but the lingual nerve does not, then lingual infiltration anaesthesia at the level of the respective premolar will be sufficient. Generally, a repeated mandibular block injection should be avoided, because the partial anaesthesia that has already set in will limit the patient's ability to give a warning if the lingual or inferior alveolar nerve is touched by the needle.

6.3.2 Indication

Mandibular block anaesthesia is used for cavity preparation and endodontic treatment, if necessary supplemented by buccal infiltration anaesthesia (◘ Fig. 6.6). It should also be used for extensive surgical treatments such as periodontal surgery, implantology, extraction and apicoectomy, where the buccal infiltration anaesthesia is more extensive and more caudal. Extra attention to the path of the mental nerve is required here. When giving additional anaesthesia, it is most undesirable to damage this nerve by pricking it accidentally.

◘ **Fig. 6.6** Buccal infiltration anaesthesia at the level of the M_1 inferior right, for anaesthetising the buccal nerve branches

6

6.3.3 Technical Aspects

Only a single injection is required to anaesthetise the mandibular nerve, i.e. the inferior alveolar and lingual nerve. An aspirating cartridge syringe is used with a 25-gauge needle that is 35 mm long. When anaesthetising the mandibular nerve, the point of the needle is placed in the pterygomandibular space. This space is bordered ventrally by the mucosa of the pharyngeal arches. This is where the injection needle is inserted in the pterygomandibular space. This space is bordered laterally by the ascending branch of the lower jaw and dorsally by the median part of the parotid gland and the skin. The attachment of the medial pterygoid muscle is found caudally and also borders the space median. The lateral pterygoid muscle borders the space cranially.

The mandibular nerve, inferior alveolar nerve, lingual nerve, buccal nerve and branches of the arteries and maxillary veins run within the space. The space runs ventro-caudally into the submandibular space and caudo-dorsally into the parapharyngeal and retropharyngeal spaces, which eventually lead to the mediastinum and pericardium.

6.4   The Direct and Indirect Technique

The inside of the mandibular ramus is more or less divergent dorsally. Therefore, various techniques can be used to anaesthetise the mandibular nerve ('mandibular block'). A distinction must be made between the so-called direct and indirect technique.

The direct technique is performed from the homolateral side. The risk of this is that the anaesthetic fluid may be applied too far medially. The danger of this is that the medial pterygoid muscle may be damaged or anaesthetic fluid may be injected into this muscle. This would lead to postoperative trismus, which may persist for days or weeks, or to a haematoma in this muscle. This has led to the indirect technique, which is performed from the contralateral commissure. The indirect technique does not have these risks.

For administration of anaesthesia with the indirect technique, a number of characteristic anatomical structures are of great importance. The following anatomical structures determine the place, direction and penetration depth of the needle:

— *The plane of occlusion*. Anaesthesia is given parallel to the plane of occlusion, approximately one finger width above (1–1.5 cm).
— *The deepest point of the front of the mandibular ramus*. If the non-injecting hand feels along the front of the ramus, the entrance of the mandibular canal appears to be on the same level as the deepest point.

🔲 Fig. 6.7   Lingual aspect of an adult mandibula with the lingula exactly in the middle between the front and back sides

— The thumb of the non-injecting hand feels along the front of the ramus, while three fingers of the same hand feel along the back of the ramus. Exactly halfway between the thumb and fingers is the *mandibular foramen*, where the alveolar nerve enters the jaw. In adults the foramen is found exactly in between the front and back. In children the foramen lies about a third from the front. This determines the depth of the needle's insertion (🔲 Fig. 6.7).

— *The triangle at the front of the pterygomandibular space* that is formed by the cheek mucosa that runs into the throat and pterygomandibular plica running from the palate to the retromolar pad. The needle must be inserted in the middle of this triangle. Unfortunately, this mucosal triangle is not visible in all patients.

With the *indirect* technique, the anaesthesia is given from the contralateral commissure, and the syringe is moved to the middle of the mouth opening while the needle is pushed in. With the *direct technique*, the anaesthesia is given from the homolateral corner of the mouth, and the syringe is moved to the middle of the mouth opening if necessary while the needle is inserted. While inserting the needle, the dentist must attempt to move the needle as close to the bone as possible without touching the periosteum unnecessarily. It is also important to hold the tip of the needle in such a way that the needle is pointed towards the bone and does not get stuck in the periosteum.

The thumb or index finger of the non-injecting hand seeks for the deepest point of the right ramus, and the fingers feel along the back of it. The needle is held parallel to the plane of occlusion, about one finger width above it. The needle point is then inserted

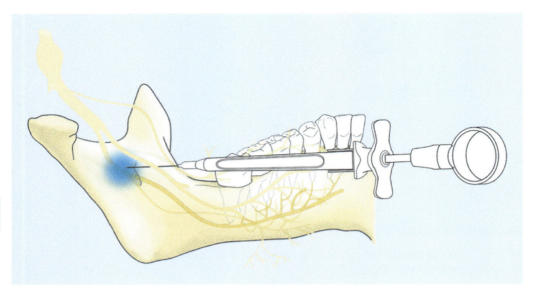

☐ Fig. 6.8   A mandibular block anaesthesia. The drawing shows the position of the needle point in relation to the mandibular foramen

in the middle of the mucosa triangle until it makes contact with the bone. Following this, the needle is carefully pushed up by moving the syringe to the middle of the oral cavity and holding it parallel to the plane of occlusion. The level of divergence inside the mandibular ramus differs from person to person. When 1 cm of the needle still remains visible and the point is exactly in the middle between the front and back of the ramus, the dentist carefully aspirates. Approximately 1.5 ml of anaesthetic fluid is injected (☐ Figs. 6.8 and 6.9). The needle is then pulled back 1 cm and the dentist must aspirate once again. The rest of the carpule is then injected in order to anaesthetise the lingual nerve (☐ Fig. 6.10).

Now the syringe is taken out of the mouth. The patient closes the mouth and is given a compliment for his/her cooperation during the anaesthesia. After approximately 2 min, the dentist asks about the patient's experience. 'Was it painful? Do you feel the effects of the anaesthesia'? If necessary, the cartridge is replaced, and anaesthesia is given to the buccal nerve, also one finger width above the point of occlusion exactly on the front side of the ramus. Here the buccal nerve, running from high lingual, crosses the front side on its way down to the gingiva and mucosa in the region M_3-P_{1inf} (☐ Fig. 6.11). The path of the buccal nerve varies, however, so that it is preferred to give infiltration anaesthesia buccal to the element to be anaesthetised.

About 2–3 min after giving a mandibular block, the patient should indicate that the corner of the mouth, lower lip and edge and tip of the tongue have begun to tingle and feel odd. One

📌 **Fig. 6.9 a, b** The technique of mandibular block anaesthesia from the left corner of the mouth (indirect technique). The needle is inserted to the bone and pulled back a millimetre, and then the syringe is moved to the middle of the mouth and simulateneously carefully pushed in so that about 1 cm of the needle remains visible. The injection is given after aspiration. **c, d** Mandibular block anaesthesia from the right corner of the mouth (direct technique). The mouth is opened as much as possible, and the needle is inserted carefully on the lingual side of the mandibular ramus so that 1 cm of the needle remains visible. The injection is given after aspiration

minute later the lower lip and tongue will be anaesthetised on one side and the treatment can start.

An experienced dentist, who takes the characteristic anatomical structures that were previously mentioned into account, will achieve a good mandibular anaesthesia in 85 % of cases. Block anaesthesia may fail due to individual anatomical differences, such as a progenic mandibula, a divergent angle between the horizontal and vertical part of the mandibula, or the absence of teeth.

Failing of the lingula is the most significant reason for an ineffective mandibular block. The point of the injection needle is then found to be too far medially, too low or too far dorsally. Other complications may also occur. In approximately 15 % of cases, blood is aspirated. It is also possible for the needle to touch the lingual nerve or the inferior alveolar nerve. In case of positive aspiration or when a nerve has been touched, it is enough to pull the needle back a few millimetres. If the needle is in too deep, this can lead to local anaesthesia within the capsule of the parotid gland. This may result in one-sided paralysis of the facial nerve, which fortunately lasts only a few hours.

● Fig. 6.10   a, b Drawing **a** and photo **b** of block anaesthesia of the lingual nerve right. After a mandibular block, the needle is pulled back about 1 cm. The injection is given after aspiration

When the mandibular block is not effective, another injection may be given. There is a chance that, during the second injection, the patient will not notice a touching of the lingual nerve, the inferior alveolar nerve or the mandibular nerve by the needle. The nerve may then be damaged without the patient or dentist noticing. It is therefore advisable to employ intraligamentous anaesthesia, particularly if the lingual nerve and the inferior alveolar nerve are not anaesthetised. An additional injection also has the disadvantage that an 'acidic environment' slowly develops inside the pterygomandibular space due to the addition of another 1.7–1.8 ml of anaesthetic fluid with a low pH. In this environment, the ionised form of anaesthetic will increase. This form is unable

◘ **Fig. 6.11** **a, b** Drawing **a** and photo **b** of block anaesthesia of the buccal nerve that runs from high lingual, crosses the front of the ramus (at the level of the finger) and then runs down to low buccal

to pass through the myelin sheath, thus reducing the effectiveness of the local anaesthetic.

Mandibular anaesthesia on the left side of the patient is conducted in the same way as on the right side. The only difference is that the left hand injects instead of the right hand. If a dentist still prefers to use the right hand, he/she must move to an 11–12 o'clock position. The left hand holds the patient's cheek to the side and feels along the front of the mandibular ramus, while the right hand administers the anaesthetic.

In some situations, such as two-sided extractions in the lower jaw, extensive periodontal treatment and (pre-)implantological treatments in the interforaminal area, a two-sided mandibular block may be given to healthy patients. The entire mandibula is then anaesthetised, including the lower lip and the front two-thirds of the tongue. The tongue's motorics remain undisturbed, however, as well as reflexive swallowing. Reflexive swallowing begins at the back third of the tongue and pharynx. Because the foremost part of the tongue is anaesthetised, the patient will not notice if anything is lying on it, such as a broken part of a molar or a piece of filling. The dentist and assistant must, therefore, keep a good eye on the oral cavity and throat.

6.5   Molars

6.5.1 Anatomical Aspects

Both on the buccal and on the lingual side, the roots of the molars are covered by a thick layer of cortical bone. The external oblique rim and the mylohyoid rim form an extra barrier for the diffusion of anaesthetic fluid to the apices of the molars (Fig. 6.12). The roots of the molars lie on the lingual side, usually below the level of the mylohyoid muscle and buccal to the M_{2inf} under the point of attachment of the buccinator muscle. Infiltration of these muscles must be avoided as a haematoma increases the risk of infection.

 Fig. 6.12   Anatomical drawing of the inferior alveolar nerve and its branches to the apices of the molars

6.5.2 **Indication**

Cavity preparations, endodontic treatment and surgical treatments require a mandibular block, supplemented by block or infiltration anaesthesia of the buccal nerve. Intraligamentous anaesthesia should, theoretically, also suffice for cavity preparations and endodontic treatments.

6.5.3 **Technique**

See the text above for the technical aspects of a mandibular block and buccal nerve anaesthesia.

6.6 **Third Molars in the Lower Jaw**

6.6.1 **Anatomical Aspects**

The impacted M_{3inf} lies in the mandibular angle region, dorsal to the M_{2inf}. This area is innervated not only by the mandibular nerve but also by sensory branches that leave the spinal column at C2 and C3 and run over the platysma to the angle. This must be taken into account when surgically removing the M_{3inf}.

The lingual nerve runs caudo-laterally from its source in the direction of the jaw and is found at the height of the M_{3inf} approximately 5 mm lingually and caudally to the bone edge and dorsally to the M_{2inf}. The path of the lingual nerve, however, shows great individual variation: the lingual nerve can also be found on the lingual side of the alveolar process above the impacted M_{3inf} at the height of the bone (◘ Fig. 6.13).

6.6.2 **Indication**

Surgical treatments such as trigone bone transplant, an operculectomy and removal of the (partly) impacted M_{3inf} require mandibular block anaesthesia and anaesthesia of the buccal nerve. If the M_{3inf} is deeply impacted, anaesthesia is also needed for the sensory branches from C2 and C3 by applying infiltration anaesthesia deep in the fold behind the M_{2inf}.

6.6.3 **Technique**

See previous paragraphs for the mandibular block technique and block anaesthesia of the buccal nerve.

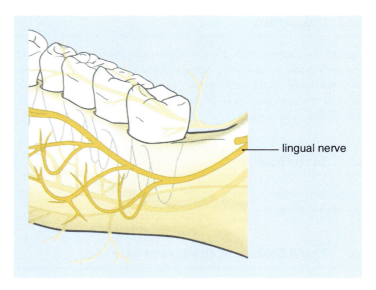

lingual nerve

Fig. 6.13 Lingual aspect of the mandibula with the M$_{3inf}$ and lingual nerve relation right

---

Box 6.1   Selective Anaesthesia in the Lower Jaw

The teeth of the lower jaw are mainly anaesthetised with mandibular block anaesthesia. Infiltration anaesthesia is only used for primary teeth and the incisors of the permanent dentition. Therefore, it is not easy to anaesthetise molars and premolars one by one in the lower jaw. This might be necessary for diagnostic purposes to identify the tooth causing severe pain, e.g. in (irreversible) pulpitis.

You can use intraligamental anaesthesia, and use this to anaesthetise initially the tooth ventrally from the tooth suspected to cause the pain. The patient will experience the anaesthetic, but the pain is not gone. Subsequently you anaesthetise the likely culprit, again using intraligamental anaesthesia. After 2 min you ask again whether the patient experiences the anaesthetic and whether the pain is gone now. When you have been able to anaesthetise the culprit, the patient will show his relief verbally and non-verbally.

Box 6.2   Long-Acting Anaesthesia as Solution for Severe, Prolonged Pain

Patients may become desperate of pain from an alveolitis or a painful, completed endodontic treatment. Initially they will resort to ordinary analgesics. Subsequently they may ask you for a prescription. You will prescribe paracetamol with codeine or a NSAID. If that does not provide sufficient relief, you advice paracetamol combined with a NSAID. If that is also insufficient and the patient's physical and mental condition is in danger by the pain and lack of sleep, local anaesthesia might be an option. Preferably you use bupivacaine, with an anaesthetic effect of 6–8 h. Depending on the tooth, you choose between infiltration anaesthesia and regional block anaesthesia. After a good night's sleep, the next day the world looks completely different for the patient.

Additional Anaesthetic Techniques

J.A. Baart

© Springer International Publishing Switzerland 2017
J.A. Baart, H.S. Brand (eds.), *Local Anaesthesia in Dentistry*, DOI 10.1007/978-3-319-43705-7_7

In dentistry, infiltration anaesthesia of the maxillary nerve (▶ Chap. 5) is mainly used for anaesthetising the teeth and surrounding tissues of the upper jaw. In the lower jaw, block anaesthesia of the mandibular nerve (▶ Chap. 6) is usually applied. In this chapter, several supplementary anaesthetic techniques are discussed, such as regional block anaesthesia of the maxillary, infraorbital, nasopalatine and mental nerves. Alternatives to mandibular block anaesthesia, such as the Gow-Gates technique and Vazirani-Akinosi method, are also described.

7.1   Maxillary Nerve Block

Blockade of the maxillary nerve induces anaesthesia of half of the maxilla, which enables surgical treatment in the upper jaw and maxillary sinus under local anaesthesia. This regional block can also be used for diagnostic purposes in cases of inexplicable pain complaints. A maxillary nerve block can be achieved via high tuberosity anaesthesia or via the greater palatine foramen. A local anaesthetic with vasoconstrictor is used, applied with an aspirating syringe and a 25-gauge needle (bent at approx. 45°).

7.1.1 High Tuberosity Anaesthesia

The maxillary nerve leaves the skull through the foramen rotundum. The nerve runs through the pterygopalatine fossa and then on through the orbit as infraorbital nerve. The infraorbital nerve runs through a canal at the bottom of the orbit and leaves the canal again through the infraorbital foramen.

The pterygopalatine fossa is accessible from the mouth. This fossa can be reached with a 35-mm-long 27-gauge straight or approximately 45 degrees' bended needle. The needle must pass the mucosa behind the zygomaticoalveolar buttress, about 1 cm from the alveolar process, and then be directed dorso-medially (◘ Fig. 7.1). After aspiration, about one cartridge may be injected. Two to three minutes later, half of the upper jaw will be anaesthetised. In some cases, the infraorbital nerve is insufficiently numbed by this technique. Furthermore, there is a chance of injecting into the pterygoid plexus, so that there is a risk of intravasal injection and developing a haematoma and 'blanching'.

7.1.2 Greater Palatine Foramen Block

A greater palatine foramen block is used less frequently than high tuberosity anaesthesia, but can be easily carried out intraorally. The greater palatine foramen lies approximately 1 cm palatinally to the

Fig. 7.1 **a, b** Photo of skull **a** and patient **b** show a high tuberosity anaesthesia. The (bent) needle is inserted from out to in, high in the pterygopalatine fossa, just by the split of the maxillary nerve into the infraorbital and superior alveolar nerves. The injection is given after aspiration

Fig. 7.2 **a–c** Photo of skull **a** and photos of patient **b, c** show a maxillary nerve block via the greater palatine foramen. The needle is bent approx. 45° and inserted in the foramen, which is located approx. 1 cm palatinal to the M_2-M_3 region. The cartridge syringe is held parallel to the occlusion plane of the upper jaw. The needle can now be pushed in carefully. The injection is performed after aspiration

M_2-M_3 region and approximately 0.5 cm in front of the pterygoid hamulus. The direction of the canal is 45° to dorsal in relation to the occlusion plane. The bent needle is carefully inserted into the foramen, and by inserting the needle slowly, the entire length of the needle can be used (■ Fig. 7.2). After aspiration, a half to one cartridge may be injected. Within 2–3 min, half of the maxilla will be anaesthetised.

It is not always easy to find the entrance to the foramen. Moreover, inserting the needle roughly can lead to long-term damage of the nerve. Finally, if the patient has a small maxilla, the anaesthetic fluid may reach the parasympathetic sphenopalatine ganglion so that unintended side effects may occur, such as diplopia (double vision).

7.2   Infraorbital Nerve Block

The infraorbital nerve runs almost horizontally through the canal in the orbital floor until it leaves through the infraorbital foramen, approximately 5–10 mm caudally to the infraorbital rim. The nerve supplies sensibility to the nostril, cheek, lower eyelid, upper lip, gingiva and upper frontal teeth.

An infraorbital nerve block is suitable for the dental treatment and surgery of frontal teeth. A vasoconstrictor containing anaesthetic is used for this block, applied with a customary cartridge syringe with 25-gauge needle of 35 mm. There are two intraoral methods for blocking the infraorbital nerve. The first involves the needle being positioned approximately 0.5 cm laterally from P_{2sup}, whilst the other method involves the needle being inserted approximately 1 cm from the alveolar process of C_{sup}. The lip is lifted with the thumb, and the index finger of the same hand feels the infraorbital rim extraorally. The needle is then moved in the direction of the finger. With the method in which the needle is inserted in the buccal sulcus at the level of the C_{sup}, the needle is directed towards the pupil of the eye (◘ Fig. 7.3). With the 'P_{2sup} method', the needle is inserted in the direction of the longitudinal axis of this tooth. After about 2 cm, the needle will make contact with the bone at the level of the infraorbital foramen. The unaltered position of the index finger prevents the needle from being fed in so as far as that it touches the eyelid. A depot of half a cartridge is enough.

The method is simple, effective and safe. However, if a vein or small artery is damaged, immediately 'blanching' and later a haematoma may occur under the eyelid, and touching the nerve with the needle leads to prolonged anaesthesia and paraesthesia.

7.3   Nasopalatine Nerve Block

The nasopalatine nerve, which runs over the floor of the nose through the incisor canal to the incisive papilla, provides sensibility to the anterior third of the palate, including the underlying bone. Anaesthesia of this nerve is appropriate for crown preparations in the entire upper front and for surgical treatment, such as ligating or removing an impacted canine, removal of a mesiodens, periodontal surgery and implantology.

⬛ Fig. 7.3   a–d Photo of skull **a**, drawing **b** and photo of patient **c** show block anaesthesia of the infraorbital nerve. The needle is inserted 1 cm vestibular to the C_{sup} right and is inserted in the direction of the pupil. The index finger of the non-injecting hand rests on the infraorbital rim. The injection is given after aspiration. Photo of patient **d** shows an alternative method, where the needle is inserted straight up from the buccal sulcus of the P_1-P_{2sup} right region so that it stops at the level of the infraorbital foramen

An anaesthetic with a vasoconstrictor is administered with a regular cartridge syringe with a 25-gauge needle of at least 20 mm long. With the mouth open, the needle point is placed right on the incisive papilla. The needle is introduced slowly, parallel to the direction of the buccal cortical bone contour (⬛ Fig. 7.4). This is almost vertical in some patients; for others it is inclined dorsally. The direction is important to avoid the needle getting stuck in the canal or having to be reinserted because it can no longer follow the

◘ Fig. 7.4   a, b Photo of skull **a** and photo of patient **b** show block anaesthesia of the nasopalatine nerve. The needle is inserted upright into the incisive papilla and introduced carefully for approx. 1 cm into the nasopalatine canal. This runs parallel to the axis direction of the central incisor. The injection is given after aspiration

canal. After approximately 1 cm, a quarter cartridge is injected very slowly.

This injection technique is painful, even in expert hands. With explanation, precision and expertise, however, this anaesthesia can also be used very successfully with children, e.g. for ligating an impacted canine or removing a mesiodens. If the nerve is damaged, an anaesthetised area may arise at the anterior of the palate durum for 3–4 months.

7.4   Mental Nerve Block

The mental nerve leaves the mandibular canal via the mental foramen approximately 5–8 mm under the P_1-P_{2inf} apices and provides sensitivity to the lower lip, skin of the chin and oral mucosa, ventral to the foramen. The lower frontal teeth, including P_{1inf}, are not innervated by the mental nerve.

Blocking the mental nerve is advised for surgery of the lower lip and the anterior edentulous alveolar process front and for biopsy of the relevant area. A cartridge syringe with a short 25-gauge needle is used and a local anaesthetic with vasoconstrictor. The mouth is almost closed and the thumb holds the lip to the side. The fingers of the same hand feel the inferior border of the mandible. The short needle penetrates the mucosa by the P_{1inf}, approximately 0.5 cm from the alveolar process. The needle point is introduced slightly medially and dorsally, so that contact with the bone occurs after approximately 1.5 cm (◘ Fig. 7.5). Half a cartridge is injected after aspiration. The half lower lip, skin of the chin and buccal mucosa are anaesthetised within 2–3 min.

If the needle is inserted too far dorsally, the foramen will be missed. When the needle is inserted too far laterally, the fluid will accumulate subcutaneously.

◘ Fig. 7.5   a–c Photo of skull **a**, drawing **b** and photo of patient **c** show block anaesthesia of the mental nerve, for anaesthetising half of the lower lip/chin area right, including the buccal mucosa. The needle is introduced approx. 1.5 cm. An injection is given after aspiration

Additional infiltration anaesthesia is often needed for surgery of the soft parts of the lip area, because of the vasoconstrictive effect. A small injection is sufficient at the level of the corner of the mouth, where the labial artery reaches the lip area.

7.5   Alternatives to Mandibular Block Anaesthesia

7.5.1 Gow-Gates Technique

Usually the direct or indirect technique is selected for a mandibular block (▶ see Sect. 6.4), where two injections anaesthetise first the inferior alveolar nerve and lingual nerve and secondly the buccal nerve. In 1973, the Australian George Gow-Gates described a block anaesthesia that is a mandibular block at a much higher level. This method anaesthetises the entire mandibular nerve with a single depot, so that an additional block of the lingual or buccal nerve is no longer necessary.

The chance of a successful anaesthesia of the entire mandibular nerve following the Gow-Gates technique is about 95 %. The success rate of a classical inferior alveolar nerve block is 85 %. The advantages of the Gow-Gates technique, however, are limited.

■ **Fig. 7.6**   **a, b** Drawing **a** and photo of patient **b** show the Gow-Gates technique for anaesthesia of the mandibular nerve. On the lingual side of the coronoid process, at the height of the M_{2sup}, the needle is inserted in the mucosa in the direction of the external auditory canal. The needle is introduced almost completely until bone contact is made with the medioventral side of the condyle

The thumb feels along the attachment of the temporal muscles to the coronoid process. Medial to this, the needle is inserted into the mucosa at the height of the occlusal plane of the M_{2sup}. The index finger of the same hand is placed in the external auditory canal, and the needle is then inserted about 25–27 mm in the direction of the index finger. Bone contact is made with the medioventral side of the condyle (■ Fig. 7.6).

It is necessary to aspirate because the needle point may enter the maxillary artery. After aspiration, an entire cartridge of anaesthetic fluid is injected. After 2–3 min, the following branches of the mandibular nerve will be anaesthetised: the inferior alveolar nerve, the lingual nerve and almost always also the buccal nerve. If the needle is introduced too far, the mandibular caput may be missed and the needle will shift over the mandibular incisura into the masseteric muscle.

□ **Fig. 7.7** Drawing of the Vazirani-Akinosi technique for anaesthesia of the inferior alveolar nerve and the lingual nerve with the mouth closed

7.5.2 **Vazirani-Akinosi Technique**

The Vazirani-Akinosi technique is a mandibular block with the mouth closed, which only anaesthetises the inferior alveolar nerve and the lingual nerve. The branches of the buccal nerve need to be anaesthetised with a small volume of anaesthetic in the buccal sulcus. This injection technique is particularly suited to anaesthetise half of the lower jaw in patients with a tendency to gag or vomit and in patients with a limited mouth opening. The technique is simple and relatively accurate. The mouth is closed and the upper lip is lifted. The longitudinal axis of the syringe is held parallel to the cementoenamel junction of C_{sup} until $M_{2sup.}$ The coronoid process is located with the thumb or index finger of the non-injecting hand. The tip of the needle now penetrates the oral mucosa, median of the index finger of the non-injecting hand, with the longitudinal axis of the syringe in the buccal sulcus of the upper jaw parallel to the cementoenamel junction of C_{sup} until $M_{2sup.}$ The needle is inserted approximately 3 cm. After aspiration, one cartridge of anaesthetic is injected. The inferior alveolar nerve and the lingual nerve are anaesthetised after 3–5 min (□ Fig. 7.7).

Microprocessor-Aided Local Anaesthesia

J.K.M. Aps

© Springer International Publishing Switzerland 2017
J.A. Baart, H.S. Brand (eds.), *Local Anaesthesia in Dentistry*, DOI 10.1007/978-3-319-43705-7_8

8.1   Introduction

The speed of injection during administration of an anaesthetic will vary among individual clinicians. On average, male dentists will probably inject faster than their female counterparts. The pain and discomfort, reported by patients during the injections, are caused by the exerted pressure, the temperature of the fluid or the added epinephrine. It is obvious that the diameter of the needle also determines the pressure in the tissues. The smaller the internal diameter of the needle, the more pressure one has to exert to inject a certain volume of injection fluid within a certain time. Many dentists assume that a needle with a smaller diameter (e.g. 30G) is more comfortable and less painful for their patients than a wider needle (e.g. 27G). However, when the mucosa is stretched well and the lip is pinched gently to distract the patient, in both cases, patients usually do not feel the insertion of the needle at all.

Administration of infiltration anaesthesia and nerve block anaesthesia is usually not associated with severe counterpressure from the tissues. Palatal or intraligamental injection, however, is, and patients will not appreciate it when the dentist attempts to inject too fast and under high pressure. The result is often insufficient anaesthesia. Not all the injected fluid will get spread into the tissues. In many cases one can observe injection fluid leaking from the tissues (e.g. an anaesthetic fountain during an attempted intraligamental injection). It should be emphasized that administration under high pressure can also cause tissue necrosis. Many dentists have experienced that their injecting hand trembled during a palatal or intraligamental injection, not infrequently leading to a frightened patient. Worst case scenario is shattering of the glass of the cartridge due to the high pressure.

8.2   Microprocessor-Aided or Microprocessor-Assisted Injection

The introduction of microprocessor-aided or microprocessor-assisted injection devices, which can monitor the counterpressure from the tissues, has solved the problem of high pressures during injections. These devices initially start with a low injection speed of about one drop per second. Depending on the counterpressure or the density of the tissues, the injection speed may slowly increase. The density of the tissues is the key factor which determines the time to inject an entire cartridge. It will take longer to inject a cartridge than with a traditional syringe, but the greater comfort experienced by the patient will definitely outweigh the increased time.

It needs to be emphasized that not every local anaesthesia technique can be applied with each of the microprocessor-aided injection devices. Some manufacturers have developed a device for a single local anaesthesia technique (e.g. infiltration anaesthesia only), while other devices have a variety of applications. It should be evident that devices that allow a variety of injection techniques (e.g. infiltration, intraligamental, palatal and intraosseous) should be preferred as they offer all options for every individual patient.

8.2.1 Anaeject® by Septodont®

The Anaeject® by Septodont® (Nippon Shika Yakuhin Co, Ltd. Japan) is a compact device that fits in one's hand (▪ Fig. 8.1). This device allows a gradual increase in injection speed in the "auto

▪ **Fig. 8.1**   **a** The Anaeject® with needle (30G, 21 mm) and inserted cartridge. **b** Upper view of the Anaeject®, showing the various options for injection speed. **c** The handpiece and the way the Anaeject® should be handled

mode". The aim of this technique is to start an injection as slowly as possible. In the slowest mode, it will take approximately 310 s to inject a cartridge, in the medium mode (mode M, auto) 160 s and in the fastest mode (mode H, auto) 110 s. One can also select to inject at a constant speed (constant modus), which reduces the time to inject a cartridge by a few seconds compared to the auto modus.

This device does not detect the pressure in the tissues during injection and therefore cannot adjust the injection speed accordingly. The dentist has to decide which mode of the device is used (L, M, H and auto versus constant). It is recommended to use the slowest injection speed for palatal injections (L mode, constant), without gradual increase of the injection speed. Aspiration is only possible in the fastest mode (H mode, constant), not in the other modes. In addition, only right-handed dentists can aspirate: the button to activate the aspiration option needs to be pressed with the thumb. Left-handed people cannot reach this button as it will be facing the palm of the left hand.

Rotation of the needle, needed for intraosseous injections, is not possible with the Anaeject®. One could, however, use the Anaeject® to replace the traditional cartridge syringe when Stabident® and X-Tip® are used to inject intraosseously after the cortical bone has been perforated. The Anaeject® is also suited for infiltration anaesthesia, nerve block anaesthesia and intraligamental injections. All needles that fit on a cartridge syringe will also fit on the Anaeject®. This device is wireless, operating on a rechargeable battery. An empty battery requires 4 h to recharge. During the injection a tune can be played by the Anaeject®. Of course, this is to be decided by the patient and the dentist.

8.2.2 The SleeperOne® by Dental-Hi Tec®

The SleeperOne® (◻ Fig. 8.2) has been developed for intraligamental injections, infiltration anaesthesia and intraseptal anaesthesia, but mandibular block anaesthesia is also possible with this device. It looks like a pen, which supports for the fingers of the dentist, enabling correct positioning and handling of the device. This provides optimal control during perforation of the mucosa and during the injection. The SleeperOne® is not completely wireless, but it has a wireless foot pedal.

The SleeperOne® can be used with any type of needle, but also has its own needles for more comfort. The device is able to detect

Fig. 8.2   a The SleeperOne®. **b** The pen grip to handle the device

the counterpressure from the tissues and adjust the injection speed accordingly. The manufacturer aims with this device to pediatric dentistry, where intraseptal injections can be performed with minimal injection pressure for a pleasant experience of the patient. Rotation of the needle, needed for intraosseous injections, is not possible with this device. The latter means that the SleeperOne®, like the Anaeject®, can be used to inject intraosseously using Stabident® or X-Tip®.

8.2.3   The QuickSleeper S4® by Dental-Hi Tec®

The QuickSleeper S4® (■ Fig. 8.3) is produced by the same manufacturer as the SleeperOne® and could be considered as a perfected SleeperOne®. The QuickSleeper S4® can be used for everything the SleeperOne® can be used for but, if equipped with the correct needle, can also penetrate the cortical plate

Fig. 8.3 **a** Handpiece of QuickSleeper S4®. **b** Wireless pedal with seven features

and subsequently the cancellous bone due to intermittent rotations of the needle. The latter enables immediate injection into the cancellous bone after penetration, without the device being withdrawn from the bone first. It is an "all-in-one" device. Injection speed is operated by a wireless pedal and can be increased for individual patients. This alteration of the injection speed should be reserved for infiltrations and regional block anaesthesia only, where the soft tissue can stretch sufficiently. This option should never be used for intraosseous injections, palatal anaesthesia and intraligamental injections!

The QuickSleeper S4® itself is not wireless (handpiece and control unit are connected by a cable), but the pedal is. This pedal has seven options, ranging from screwing the needle to aspiration. The pen grip allows good control while using the handpiece. The microprocessor-aided injection, measuring the counterpressure from the tissues constantly, helps to inject at the best injection speed possible. The cartridge cannot be observed directly, but the injected volume is indicated by a blue LED light on the handpiece. More recently the manufacturer introduced the QuickSleeper S5® (■ Fig. 8.4a). The main differences from the QuickSleeper S4® are that the wireless pedal is more easy to use and a handpiece that indicates which injection modus of the device is activated (■ Fig. 8.4b).

a

b

◘ Fig. 8.4   a The QuickSleeper S5®. **b** The handpiece indicates which injection modus is activated

8.2.4 Midwest Comfort Control Syringe®
by Dentsply®

The Midwest Comfort Control Syringe® (◘ Fig. 8.5) has no pedal and consists of a handpiece connected through a cable with a control unit to select the injection mode. This device does not

■ Fig. 8.5 The Midwest Comfort Control Syringe® consists of a control module and a handpiece with three buttons

measure the counterpressure from the tissues. The injection speed initially starts slowly and increases automatically after 10 s. The increase depends on the injection mode selected: nerve block anaesthesia, infiltration anaesthesia, palatal anaesthesia, intraligamental anaesthesia or intraosseous anaesthesia. The needle cannot be rotated to perforate the bone. The handpiece has three buttons: to start and stop the injection, to increase the injection speed and to aspirate. The dentist can increase the speed of the injection speed at any time, if necessary. The operator can hold the handpiece like a pen, but compared to the SleeperOne® and QuickSleeper®, the fingers have to be placed higher to use the buttons. The injected volume of anaesthetic fluid and the elapsed time are both displayed on the control unit. This device can be used with any needle that fits a traditional syringe.

8.2.5 The Wand® by Milestone Scientific®

The name of the Wand® (■ Fig. 8.6a) refers to the wand of a magician. The STA (single tooth anaesthesia, ■ Fig. 8.6b) and the Compudent® are technically identical devices. This device measures the counterpressure from the tissues during injection. It consists of a control unit, a pedal and a disposable handpiece, where a Luer-lock® needle can be mounted. The Wand focusses on intraligamental and palatal injection techniques, where slow injection speeds are of paramount importance. The disposable synthetic handpiece is very light, enabling a perfect pen grip as well as resting fingers on adjacent teeth. An interesting feature is

■ **Fig. 8.6** **a** Milestone Scientific Wand®. **b** STA®. **c** The pen grip to handle the compact synthetic handpiece (here the Safety Wand handpiece is shown)

that the length of the synthetic handpiece can be shortened by breaking off the back part. There is also a protective cylindrical synthetic cover, which can be slid over the needle by simply clicking on a button with the index finger (Safety Wand handpiece). The latter avoids accidental needle pricks. A disadvantage is the amount of waste from disposables when using the device. This device's control unit has a training mode to familiarize the dentist with its specific sounds before using the device on a patient.

8.2.6 **The Analge Ject® by Ronvig Dental®**

The Analge Ject® from the Danish company Ronvig Dental® (▶ www.ronvig.com) has a microprocessor that allows three different injection modes. The device can be recharged, which means elimination of one cable during clinical use. However, the cubical control unit is still connected by two cables to the handpiece and to the pedal. The handpiece allows a gentle pen grip which enables accurate administration of a local anaesthetic (■ Fig. 8.7). Conventional 1.7 ml cartridges and conventional needles fit the handpiece. The device is specifically developed for intraligamental injections, infiltration anaesthesia and mandibular block anaesthesia. For the latter application, aspiration is only possible when the fast injection mode has been selected on the control unit and the pedal is released. The pedal also allows changing the injection speed from slow to a faster mode, by tapping the pedal twice. The application range of this device resembles that of the Anaeject®, described under ▶ Sect. 8.2.1, but is more ergonomic because of the pen grip needed.

8.3   **Practical Use**

Training is paramount before one starts to use microprocessor-controlled or microprocessor-assisted injection devices. Some manufacturers offer training sessions for potential and current users to familiarize them with the device and its technical requirements. When one starts to use the device in the dental office, the user will initially be confronted with a learning curve with alternation of successes and failures. This can be understood, because most undergraduate dental curricula currently only include administration with the traditional cartridge syringe.

Many of these microprocessor-assisted devices are expensive. For motivated dental professionals, interested in administering anaesthesia comfortable and pain-free, that should not be an important reason to refrain from purchase. Once a device has been obtained, one should force oneself to use the device in all cases that require local anaesthesia. This will not only shorten the learning curve but also make the investment worthwhile.

Local Anaesthesia for Children

F.W.A. Frankenmolen and J.A. Baart

© Springer International Publishing Switzerland 2017
J.A. Baart, H.S. Brand (eds.), *Local Anaesthesia in Dentistry*, DOI 10.1007/978-3-319-43705-7_9

Needless to say, children tend to dread local anaesthesia. The dentist may deal with this in various ways. He/she must win the trust of the child, speak in a manner the child understands, use an injection technique that is effective and does not cause the child any pain and know and prevent potential complications. Finally, it is of major importance that the dentist treats the child with empathy.

9.1   Introduction

Dental treatment may sometimes be unpleasant for children. They may find it threatening; they may be afraid of possible pain. The specific dental sounds and smells may arouse feelings of discomfort. As a consequence, some children are already afraid of the dentist at a very young age. A relationship of trust between the child and dentist and painless treatment are essential for child-friendly dental care.

It is advantageous when the dental team is aware of factors that the child may experience as uncomfortable. The manner in which children experience events, the way the parents view the treatment of their child and also the way in which the dentist and dental assistant deal with the child's behaviour are important factors contributing to a child's memory of dental treatment.

If children go to the dentist regularly, their fear will, in any case, not increase. Regular visits to the dentist can help to prevent an aggravating treatment having long-term effects. Psychological research has shown that some children are more sensitive than others to what happens to them and are therefore more vulnerable to various interventional situations. They develop dental fear faster than other children. Therefore, it is important to treat vulnerable children painlessly and in the same way. This requires a very consistent method of treatment, so that children always know in advance what to expect. In order to prevent painful treatment, it is advisable to anaesthetise children. Moreover, an anaesthetic can prevent undesirable behaviour during the treatment from escalating unnecessarily. The dentist decides whether the treatment requires local anaesthesia, not the parents or the child itself. In addition to special care during administration, several aspects deserve attention such as the risk of an overdose, complications of anaesthetised soft tissues and different anatomy of children.

Box 9.1

Sander (aged 4): 'I don't want any needle'.

For small children, fear of anaesthesia is very difficult to analyse into parts. They are very quickly afraid of the whole situation because a part of it is threatening. On the other hand, they are easy to reassure and are responsive to help and support. The dentist achieves much by simply explaining everything calmly, maintaining the initiative and proceeding with the treatment. Attempting dental treatment without anaesthesia will usually only increase the stress, so that in many cases further treatment is no longer possible at all.

Anna (aged 9): 'Must it really be with anaesthesia?'

When children are older, they start to think, to anticipate and sometimes also to worry more. The dentist must then respond according to the level of fear. An explanation should be given, and the necessity of the treatment must be explained clearly and alternatives discussed, as appropriate: start without anaesthesia; then if that does not work, give an anaesthetic. The rational value of this approach increases the child's confidence in the reliability of the dentist.

Mandy (aged 3) is the boss at home and now also in the dental office. She knows that her parents get out of bed at night if she cries hard and long enough. As a reward she gets something nice to drink and that has led to obvious damage to her teeth. As the dentist explains that her teeth are going to sleep and will wake up better and prettier, her 'I don't want it' attitude takes over, emphasised by her attempts to make a dramatic getaway. The dentist is too quick for her, however, but she does not give up. Mandy then applies her proved method and starts to scream, which can also be heard in the waiting room. The dentist responds and promises to try again next time, thereby signing his own death warrant.

John (aged 4) has 'mustles'.

He can hardly be convinced of the necessity of local anaesthesia. Instead his mother says with a smile: 'You know, John, you have to sleep well to get strong muscles. Now your tooth has to sleep to get strong for cleaning and a small filling'. He agrees to that. He nods and lies back with his arms crossed. Now giving the anaesthetic is easy. When the needle is barely out of his mouth, he sits up and shows his arms: 'Mum, have I got mustles now?'

9.2   Experience of Pain and Fear in Children

Not all children react in the same way to (supposed) pain impulses, and pain thresholds seem to vary greatly between children. A toddler may fall down the stairs and, though bruised, may be quickly comforted by the mother or father with a kiss where it hurts. The same toddler may cry inconsolably while fissures on a tooth are being sealed, because the child may expect that it will hurt.

During a child's life, he or she may be afraid of a series of events. Most fears subside, because the child learns to understand the situation and learns to cope with it. Coping with fears differs from child to child and coping mechanisms change with age. The most universal coping mechanism is to avoid a scary situation. Unfortunately, avoidance behaviour is also a coping style that fully confirms the fear (■ Box 9.2).

Young children can find support in fearful situations from a parent's hug. However, they may also express their fear by crying a lot or by trying to run away. As children grow older, they are better able to deal with scary situations. They may fantasise and/or resist verbally. The older they get, the more they understand, so that situations that first made them afraid appear far less scary. In more uncomfortable cases, older children may choose from several strategies, for example, discussion or negotiation. However, they also have the choice of direct actions, such as learning to relax if they have a fear of injections or by knowing what they can do or think about in order to calm down.

Young children will relax automatically when they are advised to listen to a melody. Whether this melody is hummed by the dentist himself or originates from earphones does not matter. In the past, a microprocessor-controlled syringe with a built-in melody was available, the Anaeject®. Also listening to the child's own music by a headphone or preferably by earphones is effective. These earphones can be fixed with some adhesive plaster to avoid that they fall out (repeatedly) during the dental treatment, giving the child an excuse to interrupt the treatment repeatedly.

A remarkable aspect of coping in young children is that they do not regard themselves as afraid. One should not be surprised if a young child, who has been crying a lot during dental treatment, afterwards tells his mother quite contentedly that it went well, it did not hurt and he had not cried (!). The crying during the dental treatment was a coping mechanism for keeping control in an uncomfortable situation and much less a sign that the dentist was doing anything wrong.

Box 9.2
A child requires an approach that corresponds to his or her age, an approach that offers security and support in a sometimes new and therefore 'insecure' situation. Sitting in the dental chair, each child is especially interested in his or her own safety. The child does not really know what the dentist is about to do. If the child does know, it may often dread the treatment and will not – or hardly – be able to deal with that.

When children get older, they can distinguish very well between fear and coping. It is harder to tell from their behaviour, but when asked they can express clearly what they are afraid of and how they deal with it. They know exactly in which situations they need support, when they just need to concentrate and what they fear so much they are unable to deal with.

9.2.1 **Security and Support**

Young children look for security in new or unknown situations (■ Fig. 9.1). If they are restless, tense or nervous, the presence of a familiar person will calm them and give support. If parents or carers have had a mixture of positive and negative experiences, they often have a more balanced attitude. The more negative experiences parents have, the more they will be on alert and the sooner they want to warn and protect their child. This is the general case and is also the case for the dentist, especially when using anaesthesia.

If the parent himself/herself is scared, the child's reaction will be the signal to express very negative emotions that the parent has from his/her own dental history. The parent may rush to the child to protect him or her, saying reassuringly 'The dentist isn't scary at

■ **Fig. 9.1   a–c** Security and support

> **Box 9.3**
>
> It goes without saying that a good contact with the child's parent or carer is of great importance and time must be set aside for a thorough explanation of the treatment. Especially in these situations, the parent or carer can more easily give suggestions for the way the dental team could best approach his or her child. A positive attitude of the parent or carer is a good starting point for a favourable treatment of the child.

all' or 'The injection really does not hurt'. With this, the parent will bring out an aspect that only evokes more fear in the child. Essentially, what they are saying is 'Watch out, there is danger!' and strengthen that signal with attention: 'Come now, you're safe with me'.

Parents can be a support to the child during dental treatment (◘ Box 9.3). However, if a scared parent accompanies the child, this may mean that the child chooses a coping strategy that does not work with dental treatment being performed. In order to deal with this situation effectively, the dentist must explain this phenomenon to the parent and perform the treatment without the presence of the parent, either at that session or at the next appointment. It is important that the parent understands he/she is not being punished for his/her behaviour but that the relationship between the child and dentist will be improved if the parent is not present.

9.2.2 Preparation for Anaesthesia

If the dentist assumes that the treatment will cause pain, it is important to prepare the child, but also the parent or carer, timely for the administration of local anaesthesia. It is important that the parent or carer also receives concrete information about how they can prepare the child for the treatment with regard to its behaviour and practicality. For the child, a simple explanation is important. The parent or carer can be shown with models or X-rays that there is a real chance of pain in certain situations and that this pain may be prevented with local anaesthesia.

An important aspect is the health of the child. Most dentists assume that children are healthy. Research shows, however, that approximately 10 % of children between the ages of 0 and 18 have health problems. It is clear that during the intake of a young patient, but also prior to anaesthetising children, a medical anamnesis should be taken. ◘ Figure 9.2 provides an example of a medical questionnaire for children.

Instruction to complete this form

If you have answered the main question with **NO**, you may skip the sub-questions

Date   :

Name   :

Date of birth   :

Address   :

Telephone number   :

Name of general physician   :

Permission to exchange information with general physician

Signature parent/carer:

Medical risk from the anamnesis

....

....

1. Is your child under treatment (currently or previously) by a
   (general) physician, psychologist or medical specialist?

   YES   NO

If yes,

At which hospital?...

In which department?..

Under which physician?..

For what?..

2. Does your child have lung or respiratory diseases (COPD,
   asthma, bronchitis, frequent cough, pneumonia?

   YES   NO

If yes,

Is your child currently suffering from this?   yes   no

Is the medication working insufficiently?   yes   no

Does your child suffer from shortness of breath?   yes   no

3. Does your child have a heart murmur or a congenital heart
   defect?

   YES   NO

■ **Fig. 9.2** Medical questionnaire for children (Academic Centre for Dentistry Amsterdam, ACTA)

If yes,

Has your child ever had acute rheumatic fever?	YES	NO

If yes,

Are antibiotics necessary for dental treatment?	yes	no
Are there symptoms of the cardiac disease?	yes	no
4. Did your child have cardiac surgery?	YES	NO

I f yes,

For what?...

Did your child have an artificial heart valve fitted?	yes	no
Have symptoms remained after treatment?	yes	no
5. Does your child have heart rhythm problems?	YES	NO

If yes,

Must your child avoid physical activities?	yes	no
Must you child sit or lay down during attacks?	yes	no
6. Does your child have epilepsy?	YES	NO

If yes,

Is the medication changed frequently?	yes	no
Does you child has frequent attacks, despite the medication?	yes	no
7. Does your child has diabetes?	YES	NO

If yes,

Is your child treated with insulin?	yes	no
Is your child frequently disregulated?	yes	no
8. Does your child have anaemia?	YES	NO

If yes,

Is your child frequently tired or dizzy?	yes	no
Is there a family member with congenital anaemia?	yes	no
9. Does your child have a bleeding tendency?	YES	NO

If yes,

Do wounds heal slowly or keep bleeding for a long time?	yes	no
Does your child spontaneously bruise or get a bleeding nose?	yes	no
Is there a family member with a bleeding tendency?	yes	no
10. Does your child currently have a contagious disease?	YES	NO

If yes,

Which?...

◘ **Fig. 9.2**   (continued)

11. Does your child had any childhood diseases?	YES	NO
If yes,		
Which?..		
Does (or did) your child suffer from frequent infections e.g. inflammation of the ear?	YES	NO
Which?..		
12. Does your child currently have a liver disease?	YES	NO
If yes,		
Has he/she been hospitalised for this?	yes	no
Is your child using medication or a diet?	yes	no
Is your child a carrier of a hepatitis virus?	yes	no
13. Is your child allergic?	YES	N O
If yes,		
Pollen or grass (hay fever)	yes	no
Rubber/latex	yes	no
Iodine	yes	no
Plasters	yes	no
Soy	yes	no
Gluten	yes	no
Anaesthesia	yes	no
Antibiotics (penicillin)	yes	no
Other..		
Does your child use medication for the allergy?	YES	NO
If yes,		
Which?...		
14. Did your child ever had unexpected reactions during or after dental treatment?	YES	NO
If yes,		
What were the complications?..		
Which dentist gave the treatment?..		
15. Is your child prescribed medication (e.g. by general physician or medical specialist)?	YES	NO
If yes,		
Aspirin or other painkillers	yes	no

■ **Fig. 9.2** (continued)

For asthma	yes	no
Tranquilisers	yes	no
Prednisone, corticosteroids or other immunosuppressive drugs	yes	no
Medication against cancer or blood diseases	yes	no
Penicillin or other antibiotics	yes	no
For diabetes	yes	no
For e pilepsy	yes	no

Other...

**16. Does your child suffer from any disease or condition
that has not been covered above?**

YES   NO

If yes,

Which?..

◘ **Fig. 9.2** (continued)

9.2.3 **Child-Friendly Procedure**

As already mentioned, the child must receive information about the 'how' and 'wherefore' of the local anaesthetic. Almost all children will nod in agreement if the dentist tells them: 'I think your tooth wants to have a nice sleep while we clean it'.

Value-laden words such as 'injection', 'anaesthetic', 'needle' and 'syringe' are better replaced by terms like 'putting the tooth to sleep' and 'sleepy juice'. In fact, any description is fine as long as it is used consistently. In the same way, the use of the phrase 'to notice' instead of 'to feel' can avoid undesirable reactions, since 'to notice' is a more neutral term than 'to feel'. After all, it is the intention that the child does not 'feel' anything after the anaesthetic.

It does no harm to show the child the syringe during the explanation of the injection, but this is not essential for uncomplicated administration of the local anaesthetic (◘ Fig. 9.3). If the dentist feels doubtful about it, it is not necessary to show the cartridge syringe, as an uncomfortable explanation may have an opposite effect.

While explaining the procedure, it is advisable to mention the bitter taste of the anaesthetic ointment and/or anaesthetic fluid. It is a pity if the anaesthetic is administered faultlessly, but the child panics from the horrid taste of the anaesthetic fluid. When the dentist demonstrates the syringe, a droplet could be dripped onto the child's finger so he/she knows how bitter it tastes. This clarifies to the child, for example, why it is good to suction saliva so that

■ **Fig. 9.3   a, b** Child-friendly procedure

the bitter taste does not spread through the mouth. The pressure of the suction tube on the mucosa can serve as an extra distraction from the insertion of the needle.

9.2.4 **Warning**

The numbness and stiffness of the soft tissue, which persist long after the dental treatment, are more or less unavoidable but sometimes dangerous side effects of local anaesthesia in children. Only the administration of local anaesthesia through the periodontal ligament avoids these problems. If a child is curious about the swelling caused by the anaesthetic, it is a good idea to use a hand mirror to show that the swelling is not so bad (■ Fig. 9.4).

■ **Fig. 9.4** Children can express the numbness with the use of a mirror. The lip feels swollen but is not

It is useful to tell the child and his parents how long the anaesthesia may last and to indicate when the child may cautiously eat and drink again. A useful aid is a card with a clock drawn on it. On this, the clock hands are drawn so that the child knows when he/she may eat again. If a child is very hungry or thirsty and the anaesthesia has not yet worn off, helpful tips may be to drink through a straw and to 'eat on the other side'.

9.3   Techniques

During restorative dental treatment in children, the dentist uses anaesthesia only to a limited extent. Almost exclusively infiltration anaesthesia is used, occasionally preceded by topical anaesthesia. It seems that most dentists are reluctant to use mandibular block anaesthesia or consider this unnecessary for children. The use of intraligamentary anaesthesia is effective in children. In addition to the traditional administration with a cartridge syringe, a microprocessor-controlled form of local anaesthesia is also available, which enables child-friendly local anaesthesia along the periodontal ligament.

9.3.1   Topical Anaesthesia

Application of a topical anaesthetic enables painless perforation of the oral mucosa. At a depth of 2–3 mm, however, the needle and the outflow of the anaesthetic will be noticed. By extensive explanation prior and during the administration – 'Look, now you notice that the sleepy juice is going to your tooth' – the promise to

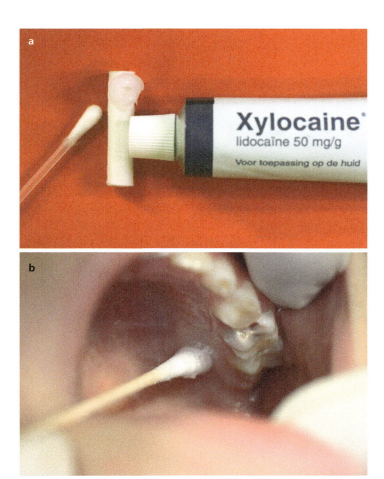

Fig. 9.5   a, b Topical anaesthesia

anaesthetise painlessly is fulfilled, and the trust of the child in the dentist will remain.

The use of topical anaesthesia can offer the dentist and child more security and so contribute to a comfortable injection of anaesthetic fluid. A choice can be made between spray and gel. The spray has a higher concentration of anaesthetic than the ointment.

If one prefers the spray, it is best to soak a cotton bud with the anaesthetic and to touch the insertion site of the needle with this. Beforehand, the mucosa must be made as dry as possible. If the cotton bud is kept in place for 2–3 min, the anaesthesia is usually sufficient to make the insertion of the needle painless.

Anaesthetic ointment and gel can be applied in the same way. Again the mucosa must be made dry prior to application. Only a small amount is required to achieve the desired result (■ Fig. 9.5 and Box 9.4).

9

Box 9.4   Colour, Taste and Acceptance
By mixing the anaesthetic ointment with cooking essences, fun colours can be made and children will accept the taste more readily. If a child chooses out of various colours, this also implicitly means that he or she has accepted an anaesthesia with an injection needle.

9.3.2 Infiltration Anaesthesia

For restorations in children in the upper jaw, infiltration anaesthesia vestibular to the respective tooth is sufficient. The bone is less compact which facilitates the diffusion of the anaesthetic. As the length of the roots is shorter in children, the needle has to be inserted less. During insertion in the buccal fold, a penetration of 3–4 mm will usually suffice. It must be ensured that the bevel is pointed towards the bone. When two cavities in adjacent primary teeth have to be treated, a single injection between both teeth will suffice. Because of the reabsorption of the roots of the deciduous teeth in older children, it is sufficient to insert the needle in the free gingiva just past the transition from the attached to the free gingiva (◘ Fig. 9.6).

Sometimes it is difficult to anaesthetise the first permanent upper molar, as the zygomatic alveolar buttress impedes access of the anaesthetic fluid. Infiltration anaesthesia distal from the buttress will usually result in efficient anaesthesia.

If topical anaesthesia is not being used, it is important to insert the needle cautiously and yet determinedly, so that the pain of the insertion is as short as possible. A certain resistance must be broken with particular speed. The needle then sinks, as it were, through the barrier of the mucosa.

If topical anaesthesia is not being used, the needle prick can be made less noticeable by slightly pinching the cheek, corner of the mouth or the lip just before the moment of penetration. The child must be informed beforehand of the slight pinch. The child is then distracted and will not or hardly feel the needle being inserted. Perhaps even more effective is using the suction tube in the buccal fold of the tooth to be treated. Due to the pressure of the suction tube, the needle can be imperceptibly inserted next to the suction tip and any spilled anaesthetic fluid will be removed immediately.

In cases of surgical procedures in the upper jaw, it is preferable to anaesthetise the greater palatine nerve or the nasopalatine nerve (◘ Fig. 9.7). The palatal anaesthesia can be given painlessly with care, especially if topical anaesthesia is being employed.

Fig. 9.6   a–d Infiltration anaesthesia

Fig. 9.7   a, b Interpapillary and palatal anaesthesia

Anaesthesia of the major palatine nerve can be regarded as block anaesthesia since an anaesthetic fluid depot is created posteriorly in the palate, dorsally of the second premolar and/or first molar. This method of administration has two advantages: more teeth on the palatal side are anaesthetised simultaneously, and there is more space for anaesthetic fluid under the mucosa in the transition of the vertical to the horizontal part in the distal section of the palate. This means that less pressure is required for the administration and the anaesthesia will be less painful. Here it is also advantageous to place the suction tip palatinally. If the child has been informed of the purpose of the suction tube, the child will find the pressure less threatening.

A disadvantage of block anaesthesia of the major palatine nerve is that part of the soft palate is also anaesthetised, so swallowing feels strange and sometimes feelings of anxiety arise. More pressure is needed during an injection in the anterior part of the palate. This may be accompanied by pain and unexpected reactions from the child.

If deciduous teeth have to be extracted, it is also possible to anaesthetise the palatal mucosa with interpapillary anaesthesia. The needle is then inserted into the papilla and 0.2 ml is slowly injected. This adequately anaesthetises the attached gingiva on the palatal side. For palatal anaesthesia, anaesthesia of the distal papilla of the tooth to be extracted will suffice.

Infiltration anaesthesia in the lower jaw can only be used in young children because the structure of the cortical bone plate is not as dense. As a consequence, penetration of anaesthetic fluid after infiltration anaesthesia is relatively effective for restorative treatment of the lower incisors, deciduous canine and the first deciduous molar. The advantage of infiltration anaesthesia in the lower jaw is that a stiff lip (partially) and the tongue (entirely) are avoided. However, the dentist does not know for sure whether the anaesthesia is really 'effective'. In strongly protesting children, the dentist can grip a stiff lip more firmly, without the problem that pain is the cause of the child's protest.

9.3.3 Mandibular Block Anaesthesia

Almost all dental procedures in children can be carried out painlessly and accurately with mandibular block anaesthesia. Supplementary anaesthesia of the buccal nerve can be needed for extractions, while the lingual nerve is automatically anaesthetised with the mandibular injection.

There are significant differences in the size of the jaw in adults and children. This means that for mandibular anaesthesia in children up to 12 years old, the injection must be given at the level of the occlusal plane.

The injection should be given less deeply for children, because the foramen is located more ventrally (at one-third of the mandibular ramus width). This is the probable explanation why mandibular block anaesthesia usually 'works' better in children than adults. Most dentists use short needles for mandibular block anaesthesia in children, maybe because they think these are less frightening than longer needles. In case of needle breakage near the hub, however, a risk of short needles is that the proximal part might not be sufficient to grasp and remove the needle.

There is a well-known preference of dentists to use infiltration anaesthesia in the molar region, rather than mandibular block anaesthesia. Research found no differences in pain experienced during administration of mandibular block anaesthesia and filtration anaesthesia in the molar area. Mandibular block anaesthesia, however, provided more effective and more reliable analgesia during dental treatment. Whether articaine 4 % or lidocaine 2 % was used did not differ in effectiveness of analgesia as well as the occurrence of side effects.

Children generally find mandibular block anaesthesia a far-reaching experience due to the numb cheek and lip and tingling tongue. If the dental treatment plan allows, it is therefore sensible to start treatments in the upper jaw for which infiltration anaesthesia is sufficient.

The technique of mandibular block anaesthesia hardly differs for children and adults. The child is asked to open the mouth wide. With the thumb and index finger, the dentist seeks, respectively, the anterior and posterior sides of the mandibular ascending branch (◘ Fig. 9.8). Measured from the front of the mandibular ramus, the foramen lies at one-third of the imaginary line between the index finger and thumb.

A slightly better grip on the lower jaw and a better fixation of the head are possible by a little modification of this method. The position of the thumb remains the same, but the index finger is placed on the head of the mandible, and the ring finger is placed in the corner of the jaw, while the middle finger is placed in the middle of the backside of the mandibular ascending branch. Working in the left mandibula, the ring finger is placed on the head of the mandibula and the index finger in the corner.

9.3.4 Intraligamental Anaesthesia

For intraligamental anaesthesia along the periodontal ligament, the anaesthetic fluid diffuses through small openings in the alveolar wall to the intraosseous space, and from there the nerve is

■ Fig. 9.8   a, b Mandibular block anaesthesia

blocked. The adjacent mucosa will also be numbed when the bone marrow is saturated with anaesthetic fluid.

The intraligamentary technique is an effective method for achieving analgesia of the deciduous dentition as well as for permanent teeth (■ Fig. 9.9). With the use of intraligamental anaesthesia, for example, Citoject® or Paroject®, a high pressure develops in the periodontal ligament. When this technique is used in the deciduous dentition, in theory this could cause developmental problems in tooth buds of the permanent teeth. If some time is taken between each 'click' of the intraligamental syringe, the build-up of pressure in the periodontal ligament will be limited. This objection does not exist in microprocessor-controlled anaesthesia. Using anaesthesia along the periodontal

◘ Fig. 9.9   a–d Intraligamental anaesthesia

ligament enables bilateral dental treatment in the lower jaw during a single session, without bilateral anaesthesia of the lip and tongue.

9.3.5 **Microprocessor-Controlled Anaesthesia**

The several types of microprocessor-controlled anaesthesia are described in ▶ Chap. 8. Most devices are suited for almost all anaesthetic techniques. An advantage of using microprocessor-controlled anaesthesia in children is that it does not resemble traditional syringes. In addition, the anaesthetic fluid can be injected with a constant low pressure, so the outflow of the fluid will be almost painless. It also avoids the maybe potential risk of intraligamental anaesthesia that excessive pressure damages tooth buds of the permanent teeth.

9.3.6 Amount of Anaesthetic Fluid for Children

In dentistry, articaine, lidocaine and prilocaine are the most widely used anaesthetics. No absolute numbers can be given for the required amount of anaesthetic fluid. Children are not necessarily more susceptible for toxic effects than adults. However, the safety margins are much smaller. The total volume of blood is essential for the dilution of the anaesthetic. In most children, there is a rather accurate relationship between volume of blood and body weight. Therefore, the body weight can be used to estimate the maximum dose of anaesthetic. In obese children, however, the risk of an overdose exists when only the body weight is taken into account. Some dentist tends to administer more anaesthetic than needed for adequate anaesthesia to avoid treatment problems, especially in children. It is obvious that this will increase the risk of an overdose. ◘ Table 9.1 provides the maximum dosage for children. The amount of anaesthetic fluid required for a painless preparation or extraction within a quadrant rarely exceeds the volume of two cartridges. Therefore the maximum dose for children is not easily exceeded.

◘ **Table 9.1** Maximum dosage of some frequently used local anaesthetics for healthy children

Weight of child	Articaine 4 %		Lidocaine 2 %		Prilocaine 3 %	
kg	mg[a]	Cartridges[b]	mg[a]	Cartridges[b]	mg[a]	Cartridges[b]
5–10	25	0.3	22	0.6	30	0.5
10–15	50	0.7	44	1.2	60	1.1
15–20	75	1.0	66	1.8	90	1.6
20–25	100	1.3	88	2.4	120	2.2
25–30	125	1.7	110	3.0	150	2.7
30–35	150	2.0	132	3.6	180	3.3
35–40	175	2.4	154	4.2	210	3.8
40–45	200	2.7	176	4.8	240	4.4

This table is based on S. F. Malamed: *Handbook of Local Anesthesia*, Mosby/St. Louis, 2013
[a]The maximum dosage indicated is for healthy children. This maximum also depends on individual differences, the way the anaesthetic is administered and the extent of vascularisation of the tissue
[b]The number of cartridges is based on cartridges with a volume of 1.8 ml

9.4   Observation of the Child

It is important to keep an eye on the child continuously during and after giving local anaesthesia. Verification that the anaesthetic 'works' increases the confidence of the child. An explanation is essential and must be adapted to the child's age. The child may, for example, notice the sharp point of the dental probe on a finger, while in the anaesthetised mouth, the child just notices pressure of the same probe or even nothing at all. It is important that the child can watch the procedure in a mirror if the child wants.

9.5   Complications of Mandibular Block Anaesthesia

Despite the extensive information given to young patients and their parents, there is a chance that children may bite their numb lip. This may cause a traumatic ulcer to occur (◘ Fig. 9.10). The

◘ **Fig. 9.10   a–c** Complications of mandibular block anaesthesia in children

danger of a bite wound is greatest in very young children and mentally restricted children. Also the time and the duration of the treatment play a role. If the treatment, e.g. has taken place around noon, children will usually be hungry and will start to eat before the anaesthesia has subsided enough. In such situations it is better for the dentist to advise the child to eat before the dental treatment. Another cause of bite wounds is that children wish to test if the anaesthesia is still working or whether it has worn off completely.

Proper instructions to child and parents can avoid a lot of problems. If, despite these instructions, the child is experiencing a complication and the parent is concerned, a short visit to the dentist for an explanation will not induce faster healing but will reassure the parent. Research has shown that the use of relatively short-acting anaesthetics does not reduce the risk of bite wounds. Use of a local anaesthetic with a vasoconstrictor remains therefore recommended.

9

Local Complications

H.P. van den Akker and J.A. Baart

© Springer International Publishing Switzerland 2017

J.A. Baart, H.S. Brand (eds.), *Local Anaesthesia in Dentistry*, DOI 10.1007/978-3-319-43705-7_10

Local anaesthesia is frequently used in dentistry and seldom leads to serious local complications. Nevertheless, it is of great importance to be aware of the causes of each local complication and – if necessary – implement correct treatment. The patient must be informed extensively and, if necessary, be reassured. The incident must also be recorded in the patient's file. This is especially important if there is a chance of prolonged or even permanent symptoms.

10.1 Needle Breakage

Since the introduction of modern disposable needles, needle breakage is a rare complication. Nevertheless, even these needles have a small chance of breaking, especially with mandibular block anaesthesia and tuberosity anaesthesia. This risk increases if the needle is (repeatedly) bent to facilitate the entrance into the area to be injected (■ Fig. 10.1). A so-called 'thin wall' needle will not break during bending (■ Fig. 10.2).

■ **Fig. 10.1**   A needle broken adjacent to the hub, after repeated bending

Fig. 10.2 A 'thin wall' needle will not break during bending. Even when a knot is made, the passage through the needle will be maintained

Unexpected movements of a scared patient, such as a sudden jerk of the head, grabbing or moving away the dentist's hand or suddenly closing the mouth, can also lead to this serious complication. Changing the direction of an incorrectly inserted needle also increases the risk of needle breakage. In such a situation, it is sensible to pull back the needle almost completely and then insert it again in the correct direction.

If the needle does break and the proximal part of the needle is still sticking out of the mucosa, the end may be taken with tweezers or mosquito artery forceps and may be cautiously removed. However, if the broken part of the needle is no longer visible, the injection location must be patted dry carefully and indicated with a permanent marker. Subsequently, the patient must be referred quickly to an oral and maxillofacial surgeon in a well-equipped hospital. In the meantime, the patient must be instructed not to talk and to swallow as little as possible, since such movements may allow the needle to move deeper into the tissues (◘ Fig. 10.3).

■ **Fig. 10.3**   A juvenile patient with a broken needle. Half an hour after the accident, the injection location can no longer be observed in the oral cavity **a**. The panoramic X-ray shows a vertical broken needle of type for infiltration anaesthesia. The dentist intended to administer mandibular block anaesthesia **b**

10

> **Box 10.1 Prevention of needle breakage**
> 1. Use only 27-gauge needle for mandibular block.
> 2. Do not bend the needle.
> 3. Avoid inserting till the hub of the needle.
> 4. Do not change the direction of the needle while injecting.
>
> What the dentist should do if the broken needle is visible:
> — Try to remove the needle with a fine haemostat.
>
> What the dentist should do if the broken needle is not visible:
> — Mark the place of insertion of the needle with a waterproof marker.
> — Inform the patient and advice to avoid jaw movements.
> — Contact the oral and maxillofacial surgeon immediately.
> — Contact your defence union and discuss the case with colleagues.
>
> What the oral and maxillofacial surgeon should do:
> — Arrange immediate assessment of the patient.
> — Arrange immediate radiographic examination (OPG and CT scan).
> — Discuss treatment modalities with the patient, parent or carer.
> — Arrange surgical exploration.

10.2   **Pain During Administration**

Even during a calm and slow injection, the patient sometimes feels some discomfort or a burning sensation when the needle is introduced through the soft tissues. An increase in tissue pressure from injecting too quickly or injecting a too large volume is unpleasant for the patient and must of course be avoided. A pronounced pain sensation is, however, usually the result of unintentionally pricking of an anatomical structure, e.g. a tendon or muscle, the periosteum, a nerve or a blood vessel.

Pricking the periosteum is usually the result of an incorrect position of the so-called 'bevel' of the needle. The bevel should be placed in parallel to the bone surface, to avoid that the sharp point of the needle pricks the tight and highly sensible periosteum and tears it away from the underlying bone. During the administration of mandibular block anaesthesia, the inferior alveolar nerve or the lingual nerve can be touched. The patient will experience this as a shot of pain or a sensation like an 'electric' shock in the lower jaw or the tongue and will react by suddenly pulling away the head. If this occurs, the needle must be pulled back slightly and, if necessary, the direction of insertion must be altered before injecting the anaesthetic fluid. Such contact of the needle with a nerve does not automatically mean that sensation disorders will occur, but the patient must be informed of the possibility and, if necessary, should be regularly checked. It is good to realise that the occurrence is not an indication of a poor injection technique, but simply a risk which is inevitably related to the administration of block anaesthesia.

A shot of pain may also occur if the artery wall is touched, resulting in the phenomenon of 'blanching' (▶ see Sect. 10.7).

Other factors that might cause pain during injection are the pH and temperature of the anaesthetic solution and the speed of the injection. Epinephrine-containing solutions have a lower pH, making them less comfortable (burning sensation). The anaesthetic solution should be used at room temperature. There is absolutely no need to store the cartridges in the refrigerator. The speed of the injection should be slow, if possible 1 ml/min, especially at the palatal site of the dentition.

10.3   **Insufficient Anaesthesia**

The most prevalent causes of failure of local anaesthesia are an incorrect injection technique and an injection into inflamed tissue. For maximal anaesthesia, the anaesthetic fluid must be deposited near the nerve or, in infiltration anaesthesia, as close as possible to the bone surface in the apex region of the element that is to be anaesthetised. In case of block anaesthesia in the lower jaw, the vertical aspect of the position of the mandibular foramen must be taken into account. If the direction of the needle is too low and the anaesthetic fluid is injected below the level of the mandibular foramen, there will be no anaesthetic effect partly due to the effect of gravity. If infiltration anaesthesia is given in an inflamed area, the local anaesthetic will be less effective due to the lower acidity of the tissue. In that case, adequate anaesthesia can be achieved by infiltration at a distance or – even better – by block anaesthesia.

During the insertion of the needle, it is important to take care that the slanted part of the needle ('bevel') points to the element that is to be anaesthetised. Otherwise, the fluid will move in the wrong direction, to a place far from its goal. Since diffusion must occur over a larger distance, this could lead to insufficient or even lack of anaesthesia. The same applies if the anaesthetic fluid is deposited in a muscle due to incorrect position of the needle. In that case, diffusion of the fluid is also hindered by the barrier of muscle tissue. An intravascular injection, resulting in injection of local anaesthetic into the bloodstream, is another cause of insufficient anaesthesia. A diffusion problem caused by a local haematoma can also play a role here. Less frequent causes are individual anatomical variations, for example, in the density of the cortical bone or divergent nerve pathways. A good example of the latter is an occasional accessory branch of the inferior alveolar nerve that first runs ventrally and then only disappears into the bone at the front of the ascending branch. This can explain pain experienced in the lower jaw despite apparently well-placed mandibular block anaesthesia.

10.4   Excessive Spread of Anaesthesia

Injecting a local anaesthetic into the mouth can sometimes have an unintended effect on neighbouring nerves. The most obvious example is paresis or paralysis of the motor facial nerve after mandibular block anaesthesia. If this occurs, the patient is unable to close the eye at will, the movement of the lower half of the face is distorted, the nasolabial fold is absent and the corner of the mouth droops.

This complication is caused by an incorrect path of the needle, which is inserted too deep and too far dorsally, and the local anaesthetic is deposited retromandibular in the deep lobe of the parotid gland. This can be avoided in mandibular anaesthesia by injecting the fluid only after contact has been made with the bone on the medial side of the ascending part of the mandibula.

Though the occurrence of facial paralysis is disconcerting for both patient and dentist, it is necessary to realise that the phenomenon is temporary. The function of the nerve will return as soon as the effect of the local anaesthetic has worn off. Because

■ **Fig. 10.4**   A female patient with a right-sided facial paralysis after mandibular block anaesthesia

the patient is not able to blink during the paralysis, there is a risk of the eye drying out and being damaged. Damage can be avoided by placing tape over the closed eyelids or wearing an eye patch (■ Fig. 10.4).

Dental local anaesthesia can sometimes also have undesired effects on the eyeball, the eye muscles and surrounding soft tissues. Such complications have been described both following an injection in the maxillary tuberosity region and after mandibular block anaesthesia. Intra-arterial injections of a local anaesthetic into the inferior or superior alveolar artery or pricking an artery vessel wall, causing a traumatic stimulation of the sympathetic fibres that run through it, may cause a spasm of the vessels that supply blood to the orbital tissues. If the injection pressure during intra-arterial injection exceeds the arterial blood pressure, the normal centripetal blood flow may reverse (retrograde flow) and the local anaesthetic may reach the orbit via the maxillary artery and an anastomosis between the middle meningeal artery and the ophthalmic artery. A vasospasm of the ophthalmic artery or its branch to the retina (central retinal artery) can lead to ipsilateral reduction in vision or even blindness. However, with the use of modern local anaesthetics, these vision distortions are almost always reversible.

Paralysis of the cranial nerves that innervate the external eye muscles may also occur. This (rare) complication usually occurs after an injection in the maxillary tuberosity region. Because there is no complete separation of the retromaxillary area and the orbit, the anaesthetic fluid may diffuse from the site of injection into the orbit. In the orbit the effect of the local anaesthetic may cause double vision (diplopia) or the drooping of the upper eyelid (ptosis), through vasoconstriction or interference with the nerve conduction.

The Horner syndrome is a special complication, whereby the pupil dilation, ptosis and the absence of lacrimal secretion are observed as a result of a unilateral block of the cervical sympathetic fibres. This is probably caused by a bleeding due to perforation of an external carotid artery branch, so that the local anaesthetic has reached the sympathetic ganglion stellatum.

All above-mentioned symptoms disappear within a few hours, as soon as the effect of the local anaesthetic has worn off. During this period, participation in traffic must explicitly be discouraged, considering the increased risk of an accident.

10.5 Iatrogenic Damage and Self-Inflicted Damage of Anaesthetised Tissues

The local anaesthetics used in dentistry often do not only anaesthetise the teeth but also the soft tissues that are innervated by the respective nerve. An example of this is the numb lip after mandibular block anaesthesia or following infiltration anaesthesia in the upper front. Anaesthetised soft tissues may be damaged accidentally without the patient noticing, either by the dentist performing the treatment or the patient himself/herself. Examples of iatrogenic damage by the dentist are a drill that shoots out and tissue caught by the incorrect placing of a hook or extraction forceps. Burn wounds may also occur, caused by an overheated dental handpiece. Because the effect of the local anaesthetic has not yet worn off after the dental treatment, there is a chance that the patient will bite the numb lip, cheek or tongue (◘ Fig. 10.5). Other possible consequences are burn wounds caused by smoking or consumption of hot drinks or food. This may result in an ulcer or even disfiguring tissue damage. This risk is greater for children, mentally handicapped and demented patients.

The companions of these patients must be warned of the possibilities of such injuries and must be advised to keep a careful eye on the patient during the remaining anaesthetic period and not to allow them to smoke, eat or drink.

◘ Fig. 10.5 An 8-year-old boy presenting 5 days after dental treatment of the right lower jaw under local anaesthesia

10.6 Persistent Sensitivity Disorders

The occurrence of a persistent sensitivity disorder in the innervation area of a nerve is usually the result of surgical treatment, such as a wisdom tooth removal. Only very rarely is it a complication of the administration of local anaesthesia. In that case, it is almost always the inferior alveolar nerve or the lingual nerve which can be damaged during mandibular block anaesthesia. The symptoms vary from a reduced or complete loss of feeling (hypaesthesia or anaesthesia) to abnormal sensations, such as itching or tingling (paraesthesia) in the respective area. Only very occasionally it may lead to a chronic pain syndrome.

The occurrence of sensitivity disorders and their duration are determined by the extent of the damage to the nerve. If the needle is immediately removed after direct contact with a nerve, there will be no symptoms once the anaesthesia has worn off. The case is different if nerve fibres are directly damaged by deep penetration of the needle or if the nerve is, as it were, blown up by an intraneural injection under high pressure. A haemorrhage within the nerve sheath, resulting in compression of the fibres, may also cause a prolonged conduction disorder. A change of symptoms within a few weeks to months, for example, a transition from anaesthesia to paraesthesia, is a good sign and indicates recovery of the nerve function. If, however, the sensibility disorder persists unaltered for more than 3 months, the chance of recovery decreases and the final prognosis is negative. Then it is wise to refer the patient to an oral and maxillofacial surgeon to evaluate the situation and to discuss possible treatment.

◘ Fig. 10.6 'Blanching' of the area supplied by the right facial artery after infiltration anaesthesia in the mandibula

10.7 Skin Paleness ('Blanching')

Directly following – and even during – an injection in the buccal fold of the upper jaw near the premolars and molars ('tuber anaesthesia'), it is possible that a sudden blanching of the skin may occur in the respective half of the face, especially in the cheek and the area around the eye. Occasionally ischemic areas may also occur in the oral mucosa at some distance from the injection point. Sometimes this phenomenon may also occur during the administration of mandibular block anaesthesia or during an injection dorsally in the buccal fold of the mandibula ('blanching'; see ◘ Fig. 10.6). Often this is accompanied by a sharp shot of pain in the affected area and by reduced vision. The symptoms generally disappear quickly during the next few minutes till half hour.

The cause is probably a prick to the artery wall, resulting in a traumatic stimulation of the orthosympathetic nerve fibres in the artery wall, causing a vessel spasm. The impulse is then carried along the blood vessel leading to vasoconstriction in the peripheral supply area of the artery. A direct effect on the vessel wall of the vasoconstrictor in the local anaesthetic may also play a role in this.

It is important to explain the phenomenon to the patient and to reassure the patient that the paleness of the skin will disappear within 1 h.

10.8 Tissue Necrosis

The occurrence of tissue necrosis in the injection area is a well-known – but thankfully rare – complication of local anaesthesia administration. This undesirable effect is mainly observed on the

Fig. 10.7 Necrosis of the palatal mucosa after the administration of an anaesthetic

hard palate (■ Fig. 10.7), partly caused by the toughness of the palatal mucosa and its sturdy attachment to the underlying bone. The most probable explanation for this complication is local ischemia, caused by one or more factors. These include an excessive high injection pressure, the injection of too much anaesthetic fluid into the tight tissue and a vasoconstrictor-induced narrowing of the small palatine end arteries. Usually this results in a superficial necrotic ulcer of the mucosa, which heals spontaneously within a few weeks. Good oral hygiene and rinsing with a chlorhexidine solution several times a day boost the healing process. In exceptional cases, such as when the periosteum is raised by a subperiosteal injection, the underlying bone may be exposed and a painful bone infection may develop. Necrosis of the palate can usually be avoided by injecting a maximum of 0.25 ml of anaesthetic fluid with very low pressure in the transition area from horizontal hard palate to the alveolar process.

10.9 **Haematoma Formation and Trismus**

A haematoma develops if, during insertion of the needle, a blood vessel is penetrated and blood leaks into the surrounding tissues. If the perforated vessel is large and the surrounding soft tissues are loose, a relatively large swelling may occur. At the usual injection sites, dental local anaesthesia has a low risk of a clinical relevant haematoma. However, complications of this kind are possible, particularly with mandibular block anaesthesia and injections into the area of the maxillary tuberosity and the mouth floor.

A haematoma, resulting from block anaesthesia at the point of the mandibular foramen, is located between the medial side of the mandibular ascending branch and the medial pterygoid muscle. This can lead to a swelling in the pharyngeal arch area and the occurrence of slight trismus. The trismus is usually noticed only a few hours after the injection and will usually disappear within one to 2 weeks if the patient performs daily mouth exercises. An increase of the trismus indicates secondary infection of the haematoma and requires immediate antibiotic treatment. Trismus can also occur if a haematoma develops in the medial pterygoid muscle due to an incorrect needle direction in mandibular block anaesthesia. As a result of scarring, this can lead to long-term difficulty in opening the mouth, which usually requires intensive physiotherapy treatment.

In tuberosity anaesthesia, a haematoma may develop in the retromaxillary area due to a perforation of the pterygoid venous plexus. Externally, this becomes visible as a rapid increasing swelling of the cheek around the zygoma. Subsequently, a slight form of trismus may also occur.

Haematomas may cause the patient a lot of discomfort and may cause embarrassment to the dentist, but the swelling restricts itself and usually does not require extensive treatment. Applying immediate pressure, possibly with an elasticated bandage, and applying ice intermittently during the first four to 6 h may help to restrict the extent of the swelling. The swelling and subsequent blue-yellow discolouration of the skin diminish slowly. Of course, correct information of the patient about the incident and the expected course are important. The patient must be advised to contact the dentist if symptoms arise that may indicate a secondary infection. Examples of this are an increasing swelling or trismus and/or fever or general malaise.

10.10 Infection

Although every intraoral injection with a sterile disposable needle will introduce microorganisms of the normal oral flora into the tissue, this rarely leads to a clinical infection in healthy people. In immunocompromised patients the dentist must, however, consider to disinfect the injection area prior to injecting with local application of an antiseptic or with a chlorhexidine mouthwash. Of course, the needle must never be inserted through an infection infiltrate or an abscess, since this increases considerably the risk of dislodging microorganisms and aggravation of the infection. In such cases, anaesthesia must be given at a distance (block anaesthesia).

If a secondary infection arises in a haematoma that has emerged during the administration of a local anaesthetic, there is a chance that an abscess will develop. This mainly applies to haematomas in the pterygomandibular space, in the retromaxillary area and in the floor of mouth. If the haematoma is infected, the slight trismus already present will increase in severity rapidly, and occasionally this happens in such a way that after a few days the mouth can no longer be opened at all. In case of an abscess in the pterygomandibular space, there is hardly any external swelling present, at most a slight swelling around the corner of the jaw. There may, however, be serious pain during palpation just inside the jaw corner. If the trismus allows, an intraoral investigation may establish in the pharyngeal arch area the presence of a swelling that is painful during palpation. Besides fever and general malaise, a further increase of the infection may result in increasing pain and problems with swallowing.

An abscess from a haematoma in the retromaxillary space can spread to adjacent spaces, increasing the risk of venous thrombophlebitis with intracranial complications. If medical symptoms indicate the development of an infection infiltrate or an abscess, the patient must be treated with antibiotics, possibly in combination with incision and drainage of the relevant area.

Systemic Complications

H.S. Brand and A.L. Frankhuijzen

© Springer International Publishing Switzerland 2017
J.A. Baart, H.S. Brand (eds.), *Local Anaesthesia in Dentistry*, DOI 10.1007/978-3-319-43705-7_11

When employed correctly, local anaesthetics are very safe agents, though unwanted systemic reactions may still appear after administration of a local anaesthetic. Dentists should prevent these side effects as much as possible, recognize them at an early phase and treat them adequately.

11.1 Introduction

Only few data are available about the frequency of side effects of local anaesthetics. Since hundred thousands of cartridges are used worldwide every day and complications are hardly reported, it seems evident that local anaesthetics – in low doses and administered with an (self-) aspirating syringe – are very safe. Undoubtedly, reactions like vasovagal collapse and hyperventilation occur most frequently, but they are mainly psychogenic in origin.

11.2 Vasovagal Collapse

The most frequent systemic complications in consequence of local anaesthesia result from emotional reactions during administration. The anticipation on the potential pain during the injection can activate the parasympathetic nervous system as well as inhibit the orthosympathetic nervous system. This causes a reduction in heart frequency and a dilatation of arterioles in muscles. Subsequently this leads to a reduction in circulating blood volume inducing a temporary shortness of blood flow to the brain.

The patient becomes restless, looks pale, perspires and may lose consciousness. In addition to the loss of consciousness, sometimes clonic cramps occur which resemble an epileptic insult. The duration of the collapse is usually limited. With an (imminent) vasovagal collapse, the dental chair should be placed in the Trendelenburg position with the heart higher than the head. The conscious patient should be encouraged to tighten the gluteal and leg muscles. If the patient has lost consciousness, this will return in Trendelenburg position in a short time.

11.3 Hyperventilation Syndrome

Fear for injection of a local anaesthetic can also serve as a trigger for an accelerated, shallow breathing. This induces a reduction in the level of carbon dioxide in the blood of (some) patients, which subsequently increases the pH. During a hyperventilation attack, the patient perceives a tingling sensation in hands and feet. The patient feels light-headed and can experience chest pressure.

In recent years, it has been reported that in many patients suffering from a hyperventilation attack, no decrease in carbon dioxide blood level could be detected. Therefore, hyperventilation is currently considered the consequence of a panic disorder. This means that the value of having the patient breathing in a plastic or paper bag is limited. All interventions that decrease the panic attack are equally effective. The dentist can 'dictate' the correct breathing rate and depth to the patient. Accurate information about the administration of local anaesthesia, combined with a fear-reducing treatment of the patient, reduces the risks of hyperventilation and vasovagal collapse.

11.4 Toxicity

It is conceivable that, as the result of the oral administration of a local anaesthetic, elsewhere in the body, such concentrations are reached that toxic effects develop. An accidental intravascular injection can cause a short-lived toxic concentration of the anaesthetic in the blood. An increased resorption rate – which may exist in inflamed tissue with increased blood flow – could also result in unexpected high blood levels. Comparable toxic effects can be observed if topical anaesthetics are sprayed directly on (inflamed) mucosa.

An overdose is usually the result of using a higher dose than maximum allowed, generally caused by repeat injections. Cases of overdose are frequently related to local anaesthesia in young children.

The toxicity of amide anaesthetics is reciprocally related to their degradation rate in the liver. Prilocaine is metabolized most rapidly and is therefore the least toxic amide local anaesthetic. In addition, prilocaine has a high degree of binding to tissue proteins (large distribution volume), so potentially a toxic concentration is reached less rapidly.

 Table 11.1 presents the maximum doses for adults of some regularly used local anaesthetics. Of course, these values must be individualized based on the patient's body weight and medical history. Patients with a reduced detoxification and elimination, like individuals with severe liver insufficiency or kidney failure, possess an increased risk of overdose. The possible interaction with other medications of the patient should also be considered: some pharmaceuticals lower the threshold for side effects of local anaesthetics (see further Chap. 12).

⊡ Table 11.1 Maximum doses of frequently used local anaesthetics (in mg for healthy individuals of 70 kg)

	Without epinephrine	With epinephrine
Articaine	400	500
Bupivacaine	75	150
Lidocaine	300	500
Mepivacaine	375	400
Prilocaine	400	600

Box 11.1 A sensible dentist calculates in milligrams

The concentration of a local anaesthetic in the cartridge is expressed as a percentage, while the added vasoconstrictor is expressed as a ratio. Since the concentrations of local anaesthetic and/or vasoconstrictor may differ per cartridge, it is necessary to be able to convert these to milligrams.

(a) Dose of local anaesthetic (articaine with epinephrine)
   Maximum dose of articaine in mg: 7 mg/kg × 70 kg = 490 mg
   Concentration in cartridge: 4 % = 40 mg/ml
      490 mg/(40 mg/ml) = 12.25 ml
      1 cartridge = 1.7 ml
   Maximum dose of articaine in cartridges: 12.25 ml/1.7 ml = 7 cartridges

(b) Dose of vasoconstrictor (articaine with epinephrine)
   Maximum dose of epinephrine in µg: 3 µg/kg × 70 kg = 210 µg
   Concentration in cartridge: 1:200.000 g/ml = 5.10^{-6} g /ml = 5 µg/ml
      1 cartridge = 1.7 ml = 1.7 × 5 = 8.5 µg epinephrine
   Maximum dose of articaine = 7 cartridges = 7 × 8.5 µg = 59.5 µg epinephrine.

This is more than a factor three less than the maximum dose of epinephrine. Therefore, determining the toxicity is the maximum dose of seven cartridges of the anaesthetic. This also applies to articaine with the same concentration of local anaesthetic, but a dose of epinephrine is twice as high (1:100.000).

11.4.1 Effects on the Central Nervous System

The local anaesthetics used in dentistry can cross the blood-brain barrier easily because of their lipophilic nature. Under physiological conditions, the central nervous system receives both inhibitory and stimulatory impulses. Since the inhibitory tonus prevails under normal conditions, an inhibition of the central nervous system by a toxic concentration of anaesthetic will

> **Box 11.2**
> A feeling of light-headedness might be indicative of a vasovagal reaction, but could also be the first symptom of central toxicity. It is assumed that central toxicity is caused to a great extent by a central cholinergic stimulation. These first clinical signs of central toxicity are hard to distinguish from a vasovagal stimulation.
>
> The excitation phase may partially be the result of a selective inhibition of inhibitory neurons in the central nervous system or a non-selective inhibition during a predominant inhibition of the central nervous system. Whereas almost all local anaesthetics have an inherent vasodilatory activity, an initial vasoconstriction may occur by displacing Ca^{2+} from the cell membrane. This has been reported frequently for prilocaine and mepivacaine. At higher concentrations of an anaesthetic, a more generalized inhibition of neurons will occur. This general depression of the central nervous system may ultimately result in loss of consciousness, reduced breathing frequency, a certain inhibition of the autonomic ganglia and finally a cardiovascular collapse.

manifest as an excitation. The patient feels dizzy and complains about tinnitus (ringing in the ears). With increasing excitation, the patient becomes afraid and trembling. The breathing fastens, the blood pressure rises and the heart frequency increases. The patient develops facial twitches and seizures may arise. The severity of the symptoms correlates with the blood level of the anaesthetic. After a further increase in blood level, a depression of the central nervous system develops which reduces consciousness. The breathing frequency decreases and may even progress to a respiratory arrest. The circulation becomes insufficient; the patient may develop a coma and ultimately a circulatory arrest.

After intravascular injection, the toxic effects on the central nervous system will manifest very rapidly (within 1 min). Distribution of the anaesthetic in the body decreases the concentration rapidly, and the toxic effects disappear soon too. With an overdose, the effects on the central nervous system develop more gradually, usually after 5–15 min. Under the last condition, the symptoms will persist much longer.

11.4.2 **Cardiovascular Effects**

Since the heart is much less sensitive to overdoses of anaesthetic than the brains, cardiotoxic effects usually appear later than the effects on the central nervous system. Cardiologists even use lidocaine in plasma concentrations of 1–3 μg/ml for the acute treatment of heart rhythm disturbances.

Higher concentrations of the anaesthetic (5–10 μg/ml) lead to an inhibition of the action potential conduction in the heart. This results in a decreased heart frequency and reduced contraction strength of the myocardium. At concentrations over 10 µg/ml, the severity of these effects increases; as a result of which ultimately even loss of circulation may occur.

The cardiotoxicity of local anaesthetics is not only concentration dependent but is also related to the strength of the anaesthetic effect. Lidocaine has the smallest negative effect on the contraction strength of the heart muscle. With more potent local anaesthetics, like bupivacaine, there is less difference between the dose that has toxic effects on the central nervous system and the dose resulting in cardiovascular toxicity.

11.4.3 Treatment of Toxic Reactions

The treatment of an overdose of local anaesthetic depends on the severity of the reaction. In most cases, the clinical signs are mild and transient and do not require specific treatment since the concentration of the anaesthetic in the brains and heart will drop rapidly due to degradation and blood redistribution in the body. The patient will be reassured, and breathing and circulation are monitored continuously. When convulsions appear, arms and legs should be protected against injuries.

In the – rare – situation that the heart contraction reducing effect of a local anaesthetic induces an insufficient circulation, the patient should be transferred to the emergency department of a hospital under administration of oxygen and, if necessary, resuscitation.

11.5 Systemic Effects of Vasoconstrictors

Signs of intoxication by added vasoconstrictors are rare and will only cause complications after intravascular injection. An increase of the concentration of epinephrine in the blood can cause a considerable increase in blood pressure and heart rate. At higher blood levels, feelings of fear and restlessness develop. The patient feels trembling, looks pale and begins to perspire heavily. Heart rhythm disorders are also among the possibilities.

Toxic effects have been also attributed to felypressin, like an increase in blood pressure. However, these effects usually occur only with doses that are five- to tenfold the maximum recommended amount of felypressin. For adults, the maximum of felypressin is 5.4 µg and of epinephrine is 200 µg.

The risk of intravascular administration of a vasoconstrictor can be minimized by using a (self-) aspirating cartridge-type

> **Box 11.3**
> The vasoconstriction by epinephrine is the result of a stimulation of α-adrenergic receptors on the smooth muscles of blood vessels. In the blood vessels of skeletal tissues, epinephrine also has a vasodilatory effect by binding to $β_2$-adrenergic receptors, which decreased the diastolic blood pressure. The strong effect of epinephrine on $β_1$-adrenergic receptors in the heart stimulates the heart action by increasing the contractile force (positive ionotropic effect), increasing the conduction velocity in the heart (positive dromotropic effect) and increasing the heart frequency (positive chronotropic effect), which can raise the systolic blood pressure substantially. Extrasystoles can also occur and, with high doses of epinephrine, even ventricular fibrillation or a cardiac arrest. A rapid increase in systolic blood pressure may result in a throbbing headache.

syringe. In addition, one should realize that pain due to insufficient anaesthesia may result in a high endogenous release of epinephrine in the circulation. The risk of this is at least as high as the risk of an (low-dosed) added vasoconstrictor. Besides, the addition of a vasoconstrictor is a protective measure against the toxicity of the anaesthetic: it delays the resorption of the anaesthetic, reduces the required dose of anaesthetic and reduces the necessity of repeat injections during treatment.

11.6 Allergic Reactions

In the past, ester anaesthetics led to allergic reactions. Responsible for this were the PABA analogues that arise during the degradation of this type of anaesthetics. With the use of the current amide anaesthetics, allergic reactions are extremely rare. Considering the biochemical structure of epinephrine and the presence of epinephrine in the own body, an allergic reaction to this vasoconstrictor seems to be excluded. Felypressin is a foreign peptide which, at least theoretically, may induce an allergic reaction. Hypersensitivity reactions after the administration of local anaesthesia are usually attributed to added preservatives and antioxidants. Since currently the preservatives methylparaben and propylparaben are hardly used anymore in cartridges of local anaesthetics, the antioxidant bisulphite is probably the most frequent cause of an allergic reaction after the administration of local anaesthesia.

Essentially, two types of allergic reactions may arise: the immediate-type hypersensitivity reaction (type I) and the delayed-type hypersensitivity reaction (type IV).

11.6.1   Immediate-Type Hypersensitivity Reactions

IgE antibodies on mast cells play a central role in an immediate hypersensitivity (anaphylactic) reaction. Patients may have developed IgE antibodies against a component of the local anaesthetic. When this agent is administered again in these patients, it will bind to the IgE molecules on the surface of the mast cells. This immediately activates the mast cells, which release histamine into the surrounding tissues and causes vasodilatation, increased vascular permeability and smooth muscle contraction. The reactions occur within 1 h after the injection of the local anaesthetic; extreme reactions may even develop within 1 min.

The clinical signs may differ in severity. Locally redness, itching and oedema may develop. Laryngeal and glottic oedema are associated with the risk of suffocation. Severe reactions may lead to hypotension, tachycardia and loss of consciousness and – in rare cases – result in an anaphylactic shock. In an anaphylactic shock, the patient does not look pale but pink, due to the generalized vasodilatation.

11.6.2   Delayed-Type Hypersensitivity Reactions

A delayed-type hypersensitivity reaction is dependent on sensibilized T-lymphocytes. At renewed contact with the allergen, the T-lymphocytes will be activated and release specific proteins (cytokines). This induces a local inflammatory reaction with concomitant tissue damage that is associated with redness and swelling. A delayed hypersensitivity reaction on the anaesthetic can also manifest as a lichenoid reaction. With a delayed hypersensitivity on an injected local anaesthetic, the patient usually complains of a painful, burning mucosa. Delayed hypersensitivity reactions develop slowly in 24–72 h, although in severe sensibilization the first signs may present already after several hours.

Box 11.4

The frequent application of a local anaesthetic on the skin may induce sensibilization leading to the development of contact eczema, a type IV hypersensitivity reaction. In the past, when local anaesthetics of the ester type were still used in dentistry regularly, contact eczema was frequently observed on the fingers of dentists and dental assistants due to spilling of injection fluid. The amide-type anaesthetics used today are weak allergens. Nowadays, allergic contact eczema of dentists is usually caused by latex gloves, composites or adhesives.

11.6.3 **Treatment of Allergic Reactions**

An anaphylactic shock is a life-threatening situation. A patient who develops within minutes an extensive allergic reaction after the administration of a local anaesthetic, with hypotension, tachycardia, respiratory difficulties and/or loss of consciousness, should be treated immediately. First, the patient is placed in the Trendelenburg position. Epinephrine has to be injected intramuscularly soon to forestall the decrease in blood pressure. Next, both an antihistamine and a corticosteroid are injected. The administration of oxygen is recommended. The patient must be transferred to the emergency department of a hospital as soon as possible (☐ Table 11.2).

Glottic oedema requires the same treatment. As long as any respiration is present, it is recommended to have the patient breathe oxygen. In case of a complete airway obstruction, an emergency intubation or tracheotomy is the last resort.

Mild hypersensitivity reactions like urticaria or itching do not per se require treatment; if necessary, oral administration of an antihistamine suffices.

Any kind of adverse reaction on local anaesthetic should be noted in detail in the patient files.

☐ **Table 11.2** Treatment of an anaphylactic reaction
Terminate dental treatment
Place the patient in the Trendelenburg position (the head lower than the heart)
The further treatment depends on the severity of the clinical signs
If the reaction is limited to the skin:
Administer an oral antihistamine, e.g. one tablet of 10 mg cetirizine (Zyrtec®) or one tablet of 10 mg loratadine (Claritin®)
With severe systemic signs:
Inject 0.5–1.0 ml epinephrine (1 ampoule containing 1 mg/ml) IM in the triceps of the upper arm or use an epinephrine auto-injector (EpiPen®). If necessary, repeat after 5 min
Similarly, inject 2 ml clemastine (Tavegil®, 1 ampoule of 2 ml containing 1 mg/ml)
Similarly, inject a corticosteroid, e.g. 1 ml dexamethasone (Oradexon®, 1 ampoule of 1 ml containing 5 mg/ml)
Administer oxygen (approximately 5 l/min)
After these actions, have the patient transported to a hospital as soon as possible. Monitor the patient's heart rate and respiration continuously

> **Box 11.5**
>
> 'Doctor, I think I am allergic to the anaesthetic. With my previous I began to tremble after the anesthesia, I got palpitations and I fainted. When I came to myself again, my arm hurt because I hit the lamp and I had peed in my pants. Never before or afterwards I had such a reaction'.
>
> Or: 'Doctor, I am allergic to that anaesthetic. Last time, and I had it more often before but not so severe, my fingers began to tingle, I got it hot and started to sweat, the world got black before my eyes and I fainted. When I came to myself again, my back was wet and I didn't know where I was, and I was ashamed to death'.
>
> Or: 'Doctor, I think I can't stand your anaesthetic. After the previous time, I had a headache for more than a day, I suffered from nausea and had to throw up immediately when I got home'.
>
> As a dentist, one is frequently confronted with a patient who tells to be allergic for the anaesthetic or the vasoconstrictor. It is not wise to minimize this and tell that this is (almost) impossible. It is better to ask questions like 'what happened exactly?' This allows the patient to tell his story, and from the description, you may conclude whether it is indeed an allergic reaction, or a toxic reaction, intravascular injection, hyperventilation, vasovagal collapse or a (known) side effect of the anaesthetic. After that you can say 'I understand what you mean' and act according to the specific reaction. If necessary, you can refer the patient for further investigation.

11.6.4   Strategy for Suspected Allergy

Since renewed exposure to an allergen can induce serious symptoms, especially in an immediate-type hypersensitivity reaction, treatment is aimed to prevent re-exposure of the patient to the same compound. However, one has to realize that most unwanted reactions that patients attribute to an allergy are normal physiological reactions during stressful situations, psychogenic reactions or the result of a failing injection technique. Moreover, allergic reactions can also be induced by latex gloves or dental materials and erroneously be attributed to the administered local anaesthetic.

For the investigation on the possible cause of an allergic reaction after the administration of local anaesthesia, the detailed recording of information like use of medication, time frame of the reaction, previous reactions and current symptoms is an important starting point. All dental materials used during treatment should also be documented carefully.

Patients can be referred to an allergologist or dermatologist for further investigation. To determine whether a patient has a delayed-type hypersensitivity, this medical specialist will apply the suspected components of the anaesthetic separately on the skin (of the back). After 48 or 72 h, the skin at these locations is inspected for a reaction. Patch tests are rather reliable to demonstrate a delayed hypersensitivity reaction on a local anaesthetic.

To prove an immediate hypersensitivity reaction, intracutaneous tests can be used. During these, minimum amounts of the suspected anaesthetic or preservative are introduced into the skin and subsequently will be looked for a skin reaction. These skin tests are not completely reliable. Therefore, sometimes a so-called provocation test is performed during which the patient is deliberately exposed to the suspected local anaesthetic. Considering the risk of an anaphylactic reaction, these provocation tests are not without danger and may not be performed in a dental office. However, it seems more practical to have a provocation test performed with the local anaesthetic that is considered as an alternative. The chance of a reaction is smaller, and when the test is negative, this provides a safe advice.

In a patient with a proved allergy for an amide type of anaesthetic, cross-reactivity can make it difficult to find an alternative amide anaesthetic. In that case, one has to divert sometimes to an anaesthetic of the ester type. Fortunately, an allergy for an amide anaesthetic is very rare.

11.7 Prevention of Side Effects

A good explanation and a fear-reducing treatment may prevent psychogenic reactions, the most common side effects, to a large extend. A medical anamnesis is essential to identify patients with an increased risk for side effects. In addition, it will identify medication that could interfere with the local anaesthetic.

Never administer more anaesthetic than absolutely necessary, using the lowest concentration of vasoconstrictor possible. During the entire dental treatment session, all cartridges used should remain on the worktop so that the total dose of anaesthetic administered can be calculated at any time. This avoids exceeding the maximum dose of anaesthetic during repeat injections during the treatment session. The risk of intravascular injection of (a part of) the local anaesthetic can be minimized by always aspirating before the injection. During the injection, the patient should be observed continuously and should be asked how he feels. In this way, undesired reactions will be noticed early. Never leave a patient unobserved after anaesthesia has been administered. When unwanted reactions occur already during the injection of an anaesthetic, one refrains of course from further administration.

Box 11.6
Some general preventive measures for the use of local anaesthetics:
- Take a medical anamnesis beforehand.
- Reassure the patient and give accurate information.
- Never use more anaesthetic than absolutely necessary.
- Use the lowest concentration of vasoconstrictor possible.
- Place the patient in a half-seated to horizontal position.
- Aspire.
- Inject slowly.
- Observe any reaction of the patient during the injection.
- Have a medical emergency kit with medication available

Finally, the dental practice should have a medical emergency kit with medication and materials to provide adequate help in acute medical situations. This emergency kit should be inspected and updated every 6 months.

11

Patients at Risk

H.S. Brand

© Springer International Publishing Switzerland 2017
J.A. Baart, H.S. Brand (eds.), *Local Anaesthesia in Dentistry*, DOI 10.1007/978-3-319-43705-7_12

Dentists are increasingly confronted with medically compromised patients. In this chapter, systemic diseases will be discussed that are associated with a (theoretically) increased risk of side effects during the administration of local anaesthetics (◻ Table 12.1).

◻ **Table 12.1**   Recommendations for the use of local anaesthetics in medically compromised patients in the general dental practice

	Local anaesthetic	Vasoconstrictor	Other aspects
Alcoholism	Reduce maximum dose		
Allergy for			
Anaesthetic (documented)	Other type of anaesthetic		Alternative: general anaesthesia
Latex			Glass cartridges with rubber diaphragm contraindicated, most modern cartridges have plastic stop and diaphragm Alternative: fill plastic syringe with anaesthetic
Antioxidant (bisulphite)		*Only epinephrine without bisulphite added*	*Bisulphite contraindicated* Alternative: felypressin containing anaesthetic
Anaemia	Reduce maximum dose of prilocaine		
Anaphylaxis: see allergy			
Angina pectoris			
Unstable	*Contraindicated*		
Other		Reduce epinephrine	
Anorexia nervosa	Reduce maximum dose		
Asthma			Preservatives discouraged
Basedow's disease: see hyperthyroidism			
Behavioural disorders Using medication		Reduce epinephrine	
Bleeding tendency: see haemorrhagic diathesis			

12

⬛ **Table 12.1** (continued)

	Local anaesthetic	Vasoconstrictor	Other aspects
Bradycardia	Reduce maximum dose	Reduce epinephrine	
Bronchitis Chronic		Reduce epinephrine	Bilateral regional block anaesthesia discouraged
Cardiac rhythm abnormalities		Reduce epinephrine	
Cocaine <24 h ago		*Epinephrine contraindicated*	
COPD		Reduce epinephrine	Bilateral regional block anaesthesia discouraged
CVA			
<1 year ago			Consult patient's physician
>1 year ago		Reduce epinephrine	
Diabetes mellitus Poorly controlled		Reduce epinephrine	
Eczema Constitutional			Preservatives discouraged
Extreme fear (for needles, syringes, anaesthetic)			Alternatives: computer-aided administration, premedication, general anaesthesia
Gastro-oesophageal reflux disease Using cimetidine	Reduce maximum dose		
Glaucoma		Reduce epinephrine	
G6PD deficiency	Prilocaine discouraged		
Graves' disease: see hyperthyroidism			
Haemophilia Factor level <50 %			Regional block anaesthesia discouraged
Haemorrhagic diathesis			Regional block anaesthesia discouraged
Heart failure	Reduce maximum dose	Reduce epinephrine	
Heart infarction: see myocardial infarction			

(continued)

▣ Table 12.1   (continued)

	Local anaesthetic	Vasoconstrictor	Other aspects
Heart valve defects (including valve replacements)			Intraligamentary injection discouraged
Hepatitis	Reduce maximum dose		If necessary, use ester-type anaesthetic
Huntington's disease Using medication		Reduce epinephrine	
Hypertension		Reduce epinephrine	
Hyperthyroidism Uncontrolled		*Epinephrine contraindicated*	Postpone treatment
Hypoproteinaemia	Reduce maximum dose		
Hypothyroidism	Reduce maximum dose		
Ischaemic heart disease	Reduce maximum dose	Reduce epinephrine	
Kidney insufficiency	Reduce maximum dose		
Leukaemia With increased bleeding tendency			Regional block anaesthesia discouraged
Liver cirrhosis	Reduce maximum dose		If necessary, use ester-type anaesthetic
Lung emphysema		Reduce epinephrine	Bilateral regional block anaesthesia discouraged
Malnutrition	Reduce maximum dose		
Marihuana Recent use		Epinephrine discouraged	
Myasthenia gravis		Reduce epinephrine	
Myocardial infarction			
<6 weeks ago	*Contraindicated*		Postpone treatment
Other	Reduce maximum dose	Reduce epinephrine	
Old age	Reduce maximum dose	Reduce epinephrine	
Oral antithrombotics: see haemorrhagic diathesis			
Osteopetrosis		Reduce epinephrine	
Parkinson's disease Using medication		Reduce epinephrine	

12

◨ **Table 12.1** (continued)

	Local anaesthetic	Vasoconstrictor	Other aspects

Peptic ulcer
  Using cimetidine or
  proton pump inhibitor
	Reduce maximum dose		

Pheochromocytoma		*Epinephrine contraindicated*	
Porphyria	Lidocaine and mepivacaine discouraged		
Pregnancy	Bupivacaine discouraged; anaesthetic with high degree of protein binding first choice. Reduce maximum dose	Felypressin discouraged; reduce epinephrine	If possible: postpone treatment
Psychiatric disorders Using medication		Reduce epinephrine	
Radiotherapy of the head and neck area		Reduce vasoconstrictors	
Sickle-cell anaemia	Prilocaine discouraged	Reduce epinephrine	
Short bowel syndrome	Reduce maximum dose		
Spasticity			Injection needles in the mouth discouraged Alternative: inhalation sedation or general anaesthesia
Systemic lupus erythematosus Advanced disease	Reduce maximum dose		
Thrombocytopenia Platelets <50 000/mm^3			Regional block anaesthesia discouraged
von Willebrand's disease			Regional block anaesthesia discouraged

Reduce maximum dose = during one treatment session, no more than 25–50 % of the maximum
recommended dose of the anaesthetic should be used
Reduce epinephrine = during one treatment session, the total amount of epinephrine should be restricted
to a maximum of 0.04 mg for adults (= 4 ml epinephrine 1:100,000 or 8 ml epinephrine 1:200,000)

12.1 Introduction

For the prevention of side effects, it is important to identify patients with an increased risk for local anaesthetics before administration. Taking a medical anamnesis, the dentist usually can retrieve relevant information about the general health of the patient. Usually, this information will be obtained with a structured medical history form, preferably signed by the patient after completion. Medication that potentially may interfere with the local anaesthetic can also be identified using a medical history form. Several medical history forms have been developed for use in the dental office.

When the patient reports a disease or condition that may interact with the administration of local anaesthetics, consultation of the patient's physician can be wise and is sometimes necessary. To obtain this medical information from a general physician or medical specialist, explicit permission of the patient is required, preferably in written form.

12.2 Cardiovascular Disease

Local anaesthetics might reduce the contraction strength of the heart. Therefore, one has to consider the risk that latent heart failure manifests itself during the administration of a local anaesthetic. In addition, liver perfusion is reduced in heart failure which increases the half-life of amide-type anaesthetics and the risk of overdose. Since the transmission of action potentials in the heart is delayed under the influence of local anaesthetics, one should also consider – at least theoretically – the development of an atrioventricular block which results in an abnormally slow heart rhythm accompanied by dizziness or loss of consciousness.

An increased epinephrine concentration in the blood results in an increased workload of the heart. In patients with ischaemic heart disease, this will increase the oxygen deficit of the heart muscle, which may provoke an attack of angina pectoris or even a myocardial infarction. Dental treatment within 6 weeks after a myocardial infarction is contraindicated.

Because pain during dental treatment induces a substantial increase in the release of epinephrine from the renal medulla, adequate anaesthesia is essential in patients with ischaemic heart diseases. According to the American Heart Association, the use of epinephrine as vasoconstrictor is justified in a dilution of 1:100,000 or 1:200,000 and restricts the total amount of epinephrine to 0.04 mg for adults (= 4 ml anaesthetic solution with epinephrine 1:100,000 or 8 ml with 1:200,000), also depending on the weight of the patient. Of course, one should always aspire to minimise the risk of intravascular injection of epinephrine. A possible alternative for epinephrine is the use of prilocaine with the vasoconstrictor felypressin, which has no or only limited cardiac effects.

Patients with certain structural heart defects and/or prosthetic heart valves have an increased risk of developing infective endocarditis, an infection of the endothelium that covers the inside surface of the heart and the heart valves. Since most injections in the oral cavity do not induce a substantial bacteraemia, prophylactic use of an antibiotic is not necessary according to the current guidelines. However, endocarditis prophylaxis may be indicated for a subsequent invasive dental procedure!

Intraligamentary anaesthesia may introduce considerable numbers of bacteria into the bloodstream. This injection technique should be avoided in patients at risk for infective endocarditis, unless antibiotic prophylaxis is already indicated for following invasive dental procedures.

12.3 Hypertension

The stress associated with the administration of a local anaesthetic and/or the dental intervention induces an increase in blood pressure, both in healthy individuals and in patients with hypertension. Therefore, in patients suffering from hypertension, the severity of the hypertension must be determined before the administration of a local anaesthetic. One can ask the hypertensive patient whether the blood pressure has been measured recently and, if so, which values were determined at that moment. Dentists can also measure the patients' blood pressure themselves.

Patients with a systolic blood pressure exceeding 180 mmHg and/or a diastolic value over 110 mmHg should not receive dental treatment without prior consultation of a physician. When the hypertensive patient has a systolic blood pressure between 160 and 180 mmHg or a diastolic pressure between 100 and 110 mmHg *and* the patient does not have other medical risk factors, routine dental treatment can be performed. Fear for the injection may induce a further increase in blood pressure. Especially for hypertensive patients, it is important to create an open and relaxed atmosphere, where the patient feels free to discuss possible concerns about the intended injection and the dentist takes these into consideration.

Pain during dental treatment will also lead in hypertensive patients to a substantial release of epinephrine from the adrenal medulla, with a considerable increase in blood pressure. On the other hand, the use of large amounts of anaesthetic with epinephrine as vasoconstrictor or an accidental intravascular injection will raise the blood pressure too. Therefore, it is recommended to use epinephrine in hypertensive patients only in a dilution of 1:100,000 or 1:200,000 and to restrict the total amount of epinephrine to 0.04 mg for adults (= 4 ml anaesthetic solution with epinephrine 1:100,000 or 8 ml with 1:200,000). Especially in this group of patients, one always has to aspire *before* the injection of the local anaesthetic. One could also consider the use of local anaesthetics with felypressin as vasoconstrictor, as in patients with severe heart failure.

12.4   Cerebrovascular Accident

Whether local anaesthetics can be used in patients with a cerebral infarction or bleeding depends on the length of time since the cerebrovascular accident (CVA) has occurred and the current presence of certain risk factors. CVA patients currently suffering from transient ischaemic attacks (TIAs) should not receive elective dental care and consequently not receive local anaesthesia. With other CVA patients, the patient's physician should be consulted if the CVA occurred less than 1 year ago. In patients where the CVA occurred more than 1 year before, a local anaesthetic can be used with a limited amount of epinephrine as vasoconstrictor (0.04 mg for adults).

12.5   Increased Bleeding Tendency

An increased bleeding tendency ('haemorrhagic diathesis') is usually caused by medication or a congenital disorder. To prevent excessive blood clotting, several types of drugs are used (antithrombotics). On one hand, platelet aggregation inhibitors, the most important are acetylsalicylic acid (Aspirin®), carbasalate calcium (Ascal®) and clopidogrel bisulphate (Plavix®). In addition, the vitamin K antagonists acenocoumarol and fenprocoumon are used, which prevent the formation of a fibrin clot. The so-called direct oral anticoagulants (DOACs) are direct inhibitors of thrombin (dabigatran) or factor X (rivaroxaban, apixaban, edoxaban). In patients using oral antithrombotics, passage of an injection needle through tissues is associated with the risk of a large haematoma. Also in patients with a hereditary bleeding disorder, like haemophilia, an extensive injection haematoma can develop. A severe bleeding in the pharyngeal tissues after mandibular block anaesthesia may cause an obstruction of the airway, which may even become life-threatening.

In patients with haemophilia, regional block anaesthesia should only be used if the concentration clotting factor is higher than 50 % of the normal level. For patients using vitamin K antagonists, routine dental treatment can be performed when the international normalised ratio was <3.5 24–72 h before treatment, and extraction wounds are surgically closed. The patient may only leave the dental office when the bleeding has stopped and the patient has received instruction on the necessary steps in the case of a post-operative bleeding.

12.6   Liver Diseases

Patients with a severely impaired liver function, for example, as a result of hepatitis or liver cirrhosis, are usually very ill. When administration of a local anaesthetic is indicated in these patients, one has to consider the reduced metabolism of amide-type anaesthetics in the liver and the increased risk of overdose. The reduced synthesis of albumin by the impaired liver decreases the protein binding of anaesthetics, further increasing the risk of overdose. In consultation with the patient's physician, one should aim for the lowest possible dose. The possible use of an ester-type anaesthetic, which is metabolised in the plasma, can be considered (▶ see Sect. 3.3.7).

12.7   Diabetes Mellitus

Epinephrine has an antagonistic effect on insulin. Consequently, the administration of an anaesthetic with epinephrine as vasoconstrictor could potentially deregulate the blood glucose level of patients with diabetes mellitus. However, the dental treatment performed under local anaesthesia can interfere with the normal eating pattern which usually affects the blood glucose level much more than the limited amount of epinephrine administered.

Only in insulin-dependent diabetics with poorly controlled blood glucose levels, the use of epinephrine as vasoconstrictor should be reduced. Therefore, before administration of a local anaesthetic, the dentist should verify the regulation of the diabetes. Nowadays, many patients with diabetes have a portable glucose meter that enables them to measure their own blood glucose level at any moment.

12.8   Hyperthyroidism

Thyroid hormone has a direct effect on the myocardium. As a result, increases in both heart rate and blood pressure are observed in patients with hyperthyroidism. These patients may also show unpredictable reactions after the administration of medication (idiosyncrasy). Therefore, in patients with untreated hyperthyroidism, administration of a local anaesthetic may cause a thyrotoxic crisis. Elective dental treatment should be postponed until treatment of the hyperthyroidy is initiated. If local anaesthesia with a vasoconstrictor is evitable, felypressin is safer than epinephrine.

12.9 Hypoproteinaemia

In patients with hypoproteinaemia, toxic effects are observed at lower doses for those local anaesthetics with a high degree of binding to plasma proteins. Therefore, toxic levels will be reached more rapidly for articaine, which has a greater degree of protein binding than lidocaine and prilocaine. Medical conditions that may decrease plasma protein levels are anorexia nervosa, liver cirrhosis, chronic inflammatory bowel disease and nephrotic syndrome (leakage of protein from the kidneys to the urine). In these patients, one should keep the dose of the local anaesthetic as low as possible.

12.10 Pregnancy

The administration of a local anaesthetic with a vasoconstrictor may pose a risk for both the unborn child and the expectant mother. Current data indicate that articaine, lidocaine and mepivacaine can be used without danger to the foetus. Articaine seems the anaesthetic of choice: it has the greatest binding to plasma proteins, which will minimise transfer across the placenta to the foetus. On the other hand, prilocaine is able to induce methaemoglobinaemia in the foetus and should therefore be avoided (◘ Box 12.1).

Box 12.1   Methaemoglobinaemia

In erythrocytes, haemoglobin is normally present in the reduced state (Fe^{2+}). This reduced form is spontaneously gradually oxidised to the ferric form (Fe^{3+}), which results in the formation of methaemoglobin that is not able to carry oxygen. Under normal conditions, the level of methaemoglobin is limited to approximately 1 % of the total amount of haemoglobin.

A degradation product of prilocaine, ortho-toluidine, can increase the level of methaemoglobin substantially, thereby causing hypoxia. In healthy adults, however, methaemoglobinaemia will only develop after the administration of high doses of prilocaine (400–600 mg). Treatment consists of intravenous administration of methylene blue.

Felypressin is related to the hormone oxytocin, which induces uterine contractions during delivery. Therefore, this vasoconstrictor should be avoided during pregnancy. The amount of epinephrine should be restricted as this vasoconstrictor also has effects on the uterus. On the other hand, pain during dental treatment should be prevented to avoid endogenous production of epinephrine.

Renal function may be reduced during pregnancy, resulting in an increased plasma concentration of the local anaesthetic and an increased risk of overdose for the expectant mother. This has been reported especially for bupivacaine.

Pregnancy is not an absolute contraindication for the administration of a local anaesthetic, but in many cases, it will be possible to postpone dental treatment till childbirth and even if breastfeeding has taken place. If dental treatment is required during pregnancy, it is best performed during the second trimester using not more than 4–6 ml of local anaesthetic.

12.11   Use of Medication

In general, many drugs bind to plasma proteins and thereby compete with local anaesthetics that also bind to plasma proteins. This may lead to a reduction of the number of binding places available for local anaesthetics, increasing the free plasma levels and thus the toxicity of local anaesthetics. In addition, for some drugs more specific interactions with local anaesthetics have been described.

The action of a *cell membrane stabilising medication*, like phenytoin (Dilantin®, Epanutin®), is potentiated by local anaesthetics and thereby could induce a cardiac toxic effect. Concomitant administration of a local anaesthetic and an *antiarrhythmic agent* like quinidine can enhance the effect on the atrioventricular conduction in the heart.

Sedatives, like diazepam (Stesolid®), increase the toxic effect of local anaesthetics. This dose-dependent effect seems to be mutual: the local anaesthetic intensifies the sedation.

Sulphonamides (e.g. Sulfadiazine®) affect the metabolism of prilocaine, which increases the risk of developing methaemoglobinaemia (■ Box 12.1). The histamine H_2-receptor antagonist *cimetidine*, used in the treatment of peptic ulcer and reflux disease, delays the degradation of lidocaine leading to somewhat elevated plasma levels of this anaesthetic.

β-Blockers interact with liver enzymes that metabolise amide-type anaesthetics. Since β-blockers also reduce the hepatic blood flow, this will result in an increased plasma concentration of the anaesthetic. Moreover, in cardiovascular patients treated with non-selective β-blockers (carvedilol, labetalol, oxprenolol, pindolol, propranolol and sotalol), epinephrine may lead to hypertension. In these patients, the blockade of the β_2-receptors prevents the vasodilatation in skeletal muscles that compensates the α-adrenergic vasoconstriction. This risk does not occur with selective β-blockers (atenolol, betaxolol, bisoprolol, celiprolol, esmolol, metoprolol and nebivolol).

Tricyclic antidepressants (e.g. amitriptyline, clomipramine) inhibit the reuptake of epinephrine into nerve cells, which increases the concentration at the site of the receptor. Consequently, tricyclic antidepressants can potentially potentiate the cardio-vascular effects of epinephrine. Therefore, in these patients the use of epinephrine as vasoconstrictor is discouraged. Other anti-depressants, the so-called monoamine oxidase inhibitors (MAO inhibitors, e.g. moclobemide), inhibit the degradation of epinephrine in the central nervous system so that simultaneous use of epinephrine likewise increases the risk of a hypertensive reaction.

Phenothiazines (antipsychotics, like chlorpromazine and perphenazine) block the α-adrenergic receptors. In these patients, administration of epinephrine may lead to a serious fall of the blood pressure: the α-adrenergic vasoconstriction cannot occur, yet the β_2-adrenergic vasodilatation will take place. Therefore, epinephrine should not be used as vasoconstrictor in patients using phenothiazines.

One also has to be careful with patients using *nose drops*. Nose drops sometimes contain the sympathicomimetic compound phenylephrine, causing unexpected strong effects of epinephrine. *Cocaine* and derivatives like 'crack' are sympathicomimetics too. Therefore, epinephrine is contraindicated as vasoconstrictor for individuals who recently used cocaine.

12

Legal Aspects of Local Anaesthesia

W.G. Brands

© Springer International Publishing Switzerland 2017
J.A. Baart, H.S. Brand (eds.), *Local Anaesthesia in Dentistry*, DOI 10.1007/978-3-319-43705-7_13

The dentist should consider the possibility that, in certain cases, he/she may be asked to justify giving or permitting the application of local anaesthesia before a court. Verdicts, and the laws on which they are based, differ from country to country and often even differ within a country, e.g. within the United States, Canada and Australia. It is necessary to keep in mind that a dentist is only subject to the law of the country, province or state in which he/she is currently practising. Despite this variance, there are many similarities between the various jurisdictions. Therefore, comments on the legal aspects of the use of local anaesthetics in dentistry often have international value.

A dentist may be summoned before various judges, each of whom will consider the case according to his or her own criteria. For this reason, first the different courts that may judge a dentist's case are described in this chapter. Subsequently, the competency of the dentist and co-workers with regard to the administration of local anaesthesia is discussed. Following this, several cases illustrate the kind of legal problems a dentist may be confronted with after applying local anaesthesia and the circumstances under which the dentist may be held to account. Finally, suggestions are given of how to reduce the risk of juridical problems after the administration of local anaesthesia.

13.1 Judges and Courts

If a patient believes he or she has been treated unjustly by his/her dentist, the patient may file a formal complaint to various courts. The patient's choice of the different courts will usually be influenced by two considerations:

- How simple and expensive is the legal procedure?
- What will I gain from the procedure?

Usually, the complainant hopes that the accused dentist will receive a form of punishment or caution and that the damage suffered will be compensated. Depending on his/her aim, the patient may approach the following judges or courts:

1. *The disciplinary board*. Applying to this board is generally a free procedure. The court considers whether disciplinary measures should be imposed on the dentist, and these measures may vary from a caution to prohibiting the dentist from practising. For the dentist, this legal proceeding is very unpleasant, not only because of the potential punitive measures but also because of the publicity. Many dental boards publish the names of the involved dentists online, especially in cases of a suspension or a permanent prohibition to practise dentistry. Some boards even provide complete case files, including the dentist's full name, for public inspection.

Such boards include the General Dental Council in Great Britain (▶ http://www.gdc-uk.org) and disciplinary councils in Colorado (USA) (▶ http://www.dora.state.co.us/DENTAL/) and New Zealand (▶ http://www.dcnz.org.nz/).

2. *The criminal court.* By submitting a complaint, the patient starts a procedure which may eventually lead to the prosecution of the dentist according to the criminal law. Because criminal law is regarded as an utmost serious measure, dentists rarely are confronted with the criminal court. However, if a patient should die after administration of local anaesthesia, a criminal law procedure is nowadays likely. For the average law-abiding dentist, a criminal law procedure and certainly a consequent prison sentence will be quite a traumatic experience. In the United States and countries within the Commonwealth, often a disciplinary procedure will be started automatically against dentists who are convicted according to criminal law, often without the involvement of the respective patient.

3. *The civil law court.* If a patient has suffered damage for which the dentist is responsible, the patient may summon the dentist before a civil law court. The procedure usually follows in writing. Though the civil judge gives a verdict concerning the damages of the patient, this verdict in most cases does not include any penalty. A disadvantage for the dentist is that a civil law case is often very expensive. The compensation to be paid can reach incredible proportions, especially in the United States. This usually concerns cases where the dentist's reckless treatment has led to permanent medical damage to the patient. In the United States, in such cases so-called punitive damages may be imposed. In countries of the Commonwealth, this compensation is called an exemplary damage award. The following case from New Zealand demonstrates that there are very strict grounds upon which punitive damage is awarded.

■ **Case: Punitive Damage in Dentistry**

(NZCA 215, 1999, New Zealand)

During endodontic treatment, a part of an endodontic instrument remained in the patient's root canal. The patient claimed she suffered from periodic inflammation and pain. Allegations relate to the original treatment and failure to notice that the instrument had fractured, with part remaining in the tooth, the failure to discover or disclose the presence of the fragment and to take steps to relieve the pain, and generally acting in a high-handed manner by never admitting the negligent conduct or offering assistance. It is alleged that these matters were aggravated by oppressive tactics adopted by the dentist after notice had been given of the intention to take proceedings. The claim was for exemplary damages of $250,000.

The court stated about the exemplary damages: 'The indications from the evidence presently available consist more with the dentist not having discovered the fragment. Mrs X confirmed that this is the allegation. It may be a case of negligence but not of a kind that would attract exemplary damages. Failure by a medical or dental caregiver to investigate a suspected cause of persistent pain or discomfort, though negligent, would be likely to attract an award of exemplary damages only where the dentist is shown to had improper motive, reckless disregard for the patient's health or safety, or some special flagrancy reflecting the type of conduct that amounts to an affront to the community. It is not enough to simply allege that the caregiver is high-handed. This case involves allegations of negligence that may be possible to prove but it is not sufficient to be one of those rare cases in which exemplary damages might be awarded'.

In a study by Cohen [2], it appeared that the median amount for punitive damage was US \$187,000, with a peak of \$75 million. Punitive damage is usually awarded in cases relating to general medical practice; very rarely is it awarded in dentistry cases.

One difference between disciplinary and criminal law on the one hand and civil law on the other hand is especially significant for dental practices where many treatments are delegated to an employee. The disciplinary and criminal courts are only interested in whether the dentist himself/herself is to blame. The reproach may be that the dentist himself/herself has been insufficiently cautious in the application of local anaesthesia, but also that he/she has delegated the application incorrectly. One can, however, also approach a civil law court if the dentist is not personally to blame, but rather one of his/her staff.

13.2 Competency to Give Local Anaesthesia

The competencies of medical professionals are generally described in a law that governs the medical professions. A special law for dentistry, a Dental Practice Act, is not uncommon. Often these laws are relatively general and are implemented following the guidelines of the dental boards or of the national dental practitioners' organisation.

13.2.1 General and Local Anaesthesia Given by the Dentist

In almost all countries, giving anaesthesia is considered a relatively hazardous procedure that may not be performed by just anyone. In some cases the law appears to regard anaesthesia as more dangerous than, for instance, an extraction. Article 139 A of the

Dental Practitioners Registration Act (2001) in Queensland (Australia), for example, states that in an emergency, an unqualified person may extract a tooth in the absence of a dentist but cannot give a local anaesthetic.

Usually a distinction is made between giving local anaesthesia and general anaesthesia. On the basis of the dentist's education, or in many states on the basis of his/her licence, a dentist is generally qualified to administer a local anaesthetic. An additional licence is usually required for giving general anaesthesia, and special conditions are required for the dental practice. For example, the guidelines for giving general anaesthesia in Ontario (Canada) demand that the dentist has followed a course on narcosis and sedation which shows that he/she is capable of giving general anaesthesia. In some countries, such as the Netherlands, there is no obligation to obtain a separate certificate, but the dentist must demonstrate with a course diploma that he/she is skilled in giving (local) anaesthesia. In practice, the two systems do not differ greatly.

13.2.2 Local Anaesthesia Given by Paramedics

Worldwide there are various paramedics active in dental practice. Because their titles and corresponding qualifications differ from country to country, this section will explore the main professionals involved: the dental assistant, the dental hygienist and the dental therapist.

The dental assistant has a relatively low level of dental education and in most countries is not qualified to give local anaesthesia. In some countries an exception is made with regard to the application of topical anaesthesia. In the state of Montana (USA), for example, a dental assistant may apply topical anaesthesia under the direct supervision of a dentist (Montana, Board of Dentistry rule 24.138.406). The Netherlands provides an exception to this point; since in this country a dental assistant is permitted to give infiltration anaesthesia provided that a dentist has given the order, the assistant is competent, and there is a form of supervision (Article 38 BIG). A Dutch dentist must be able to demonstrate that all conditions have been met. If this is not the case, both the assistant and the dentist may face a jail sentence. With such measures, the Dutch authorities try to prevent unqualified dental assistants from giving local anaesthesia.

The conditions under which *dental hygienists* may administer local anaesthetics vary widely internationally. In the Netherlands, a dental hygienist is qualified to give local anaesthesia for dental treatments, even in the absence of the dentist. In most other countries, a dental hygienist is only permitted to give local anaesthesia under supervision. If this requirement is not met, disciplinary measures will follow.

Some jurisdictions, such as African countries and Canadian and Australian provinces, also recognise the *dental therapist*. In the United States, Minnesota claims to be the first state that established licensure of dental therapists. The dental therapist has more extensive qualifications than the dental hygienist, including being qualified to administer local anaesthesia.

■ **Case: Unqualified Application of a Mandibular Block**
(South Carolina State Board of Dentistry, USA)
A dentist permitted his dental hygienist to give a mandibular block without the required supervision. In principle, this would result in a suspension of his licence for 5 years. He agreed with the dental board, however, that he would pay a fine of US $3000, follow a course in ethics and would redo his exam in jurisprudence. Furthermore, he would pay utmost attention that insufficiently qualified staff would no longer perform treatments in his practice.

13.3 Liability

There are only a few cases known where the administration of a local anaesthetic has led to a complaint or claim. In the following section, various situations will be discussed in which the administration of a local anaesthetic has led to legal proceedings. The reader must bear in mind that jurisprudence in one country does not automatically apply to dental practices in other countries. Nevertheless, the cases presented provide a reasonable overview of what a dentist may be blamed for by a patient if the administration of anaesthesia does not go according to plan.

13.3.1 A Damaged Nerve Following Anaesthesia: Informed Consent

■ **Case: Nerve Damage Following a Mandibular Block**
(Dental Board Utrecht, the Netherlands)
A patient retained a partly anaesthetised tongue following a mandibular block. The anaesthesia was given for soft tissue treatment. When asked, the dentist explained that the nerve had been touched during the anaesthesia, but that the symptoms would most likely disappear. However, the symptoms did not disappear and the patient pressed charges. The patient based his complaint on the fact that prior to the treatment, the dentist had given insufficient information regarding the possible risks. The patient explained that loss of feeling in the tongue significantly hindered his eating and his social life. He also suffered from insomnia and headaches. The dental board judged that the dentist

could not be blamed for pricking the lingual nerve and that there is a consensus within the profession that patients do not need to be informed of very rare risks. The charge was dismissed.

In the above-mentioned case, the complaint was rejected because the risk of the particular complication was very small. According to the available literature, the incidence of permanent damage to the lingual nerve as a result of anaesthesia varies between 1 in 26,000 and 1 in 800,000 [5]. If transient sensitivity disorders are included, the incidence increases to 1 in 2667 [6].

The dental board assumed in the above case that the dentist was not required to warn the patient on the basis of the risk being so small. The disciplinary court took as a starting point for their judgement the fact that the dentist was reasonable, competent and well-practising. In various countries, such as Great Britain, Canada, the Netherlands and some states of the United States, it counts not only whether or not a reasonable practising dentist should have warned the patient of this risk but also whether or not a reasonable patient would have refused anaesthesia in the same situation if he/she had been sufficiently informed [1]. In answer to the last question, the following factors will be of importance:

- What was the risk that the complication might occur?
- How would the situation have developed without treatment?
- Could other, less risky treatment methods have been employed? If so, what was the chance of success of such treatment?
- How serious was the complication?

The above requirements are interdependent. A sensible patient will take a relatively large risk for a life-saving operation. On the other hand, a patient will hardly accept any risk for cosmetic surgery. If we apply these principles to the question of whether a patient must be informed of certain risks of local anaesthesia, we must make the following considerations.

Damage to a nerve may be hardly invalidating or life-threatening, but it does cause particular discomfort. The risk of damage to a nerve as a result of the administration of local anaesthesia is, however, so small that a reasonable patient will easily agree to anaesthesia for necessary dental treatment.

The situation is different if the patient's health will not be damaged in any way when he or she refrains from treatment, for example, if the treatment is required simply for cosmetic reasons. Imagine that the dentist from the case above had administered local anaesthesia to replace an amalgam restoration with a composite white filling for cosmetic reasons. In this case it is questionable whether a reasonable patient will regard the small risk as acceptable.

Finally, a reasonable patient would not have accepted any risks at all if less risky alternatives were available. In that case the question is why the dentist has not considered, for example, the use of intraligamentary anaesthesia instead of mandibular block anaesthesia [3]. If an anaesthetic technique is available that reduces the chance of nerve damage, the dentist has a greater obligation to inform the patient sufficiently when he/she chooses the more risky injection technique.

When a dentist knows more about a patient, the reasonable patient becomes less abstract and the dentist may decide differently. For example, patients who have to speak a lot in their profession will be less willing to accept a permanently anaesthetised lip than someone who works with his or her hands. This means that, when giving anaesthesia, the dentist should warn a singer more readily and extensively of the risks of sensitivity disorders than, for example, a car mechanic.

Another question is whether informed consent for giving local anaesthesia should be obtained verbally or in writing. Legislation on this point varies widely, so that nothing much helpful can be said about it globally. Otherwise, the general consensus worldwide is that a dentist must be able to demonstrate the informed consent. Written permission by the patient can therefore also be very useful in jurisdictions where dentists are not obliged to obtain written informed consent. An American study has shown that dental specialists usually record written informed consent, while general dental practitioners obtain written informed consent less frequently [4].

13.3.2   No Anaesthesia Given, Faulty Injection or Insufficient Anaesthesia

For children, anaesthesia can often be a necessity. A very far-reaching verdict was given by the Dentistry Examining Board of Wisconsin (USA) in the following case.

■ **Case: Treatment of Children Without Anaesthesia**
(Wisconsin Court of Appeals 02–2218, USA)
A dentist treated dental caries in four children under the age of 3 years. He did not use anaesthesia nor did he inform the parents of the options for the administration of anaesthesia. After charges had been pressed, the dental board determined that the treatment of two children had been substandard. The board reprimanded the dentist and limited his licence to the treatment of children over 14 years old. The board also obliged him to attend a course in pain control.

A similar verdict – though in a case involving an adult – was pronounced by the Professional Conduct Committee (PCC) of the General Dental Council (GDC) in Great Britain.

- **Case: Treatment of Adults Without Anaesthesia**

(Professional Conduct Committee, Great Britain)
A dentist began a root canal treatment. He did not perform a sensitivity test and started to drill without giving anaesthesia. The PCC judged that without a sensitivity test, the dentist could not know whether the tooth was vital or not and therefore should not have performed the treatment without anaesthesia or without explanation to the patient that the treatment could be painful. In this case the PCC judged it necessary that permission from the patient should have been obtained before drilling without anaesthesia.

The above cases concerned not giving anaesthesia; it is clear that the option of anaesthesia must, in any case, be offered to the patient. If subsequently anaesthesia is given, the dentist must observe the patient's behaviour very well to ascertain whether anything is wrong.

- **Case: The Patient Indicates During the Injection That Something Is Wrong**

(Professional Conduct Committee, Great Britain)
Charges were pressed against a dentist for several matters concerning practice and incorrect treatments. One of the charges concerned the administration of anaesthesia. In the first place, the dentist was blamed for giving anaesthesia without obtaining informed consent. During the administration of anaesthesia, the dentist perforated the nose floor and injected the anaesthetic into the nasal cavity. The charge was not only that the dentist had perforated the nose floor but also that the dentist continued with the treatment when the patient indicated that something was wrong during the administration of anaesthesia.

The Conduct Committee concluded that the dentist's knowledge was lacking in a number of areas and that these flaws needed to be corrected.

The patient's behaviour may also be important once the actual treatment has commenced and the patient indicates that the anaesthesia is not working.

- **Case: The Patient Indicates That the Anaesthesia Is Not Working**

(Disciplinary Court, the Netherlands)
A patient was receiving a number of dental implants, for which anaesthesia had been administered. The anaesthesia worked for about 40 min. Although the anaesthesia had lost its effect, the dentist continued with the treatment because it was not yet completely finished. The patient subsequently lodged a complaint against the dentist, partly because of the painful treatment. The

disciplinary court judged concerning the anaesthesia that it had been perfectly possible to give an additional amount of anaesthetic and that the dentist had been wrong not to do so. Because the disciplinary court also doubted the necessity for the implants, the dentist was given a caution.

In this case, the administration of an additional amount of anaesthesia had been possible. There are also cases where a local anaesthetic that has been applied correctly is not sufficiently effective, for example, in certain forms of pulpitis. In such cases it is particularly important to inform the patient correctly. If there is a moderate chance that the patient cannot be fully anaesthetised, it is reasonable to assume the patient may refuse to give permission. If a dentist cannot convince the patient that the treatment should nevertheless be performed, it must be postponed. There may also be cases where the patient thinks he or she feels something during the treatment. In this case the dentist should give additional anaesthesia. If this is not successful, the dentist must consider whether the treatment can be halted or whether a 'point of no return' has been passed. In the latter case, the dentist could proceed with the treatment until a moment is reached where the situation is stable again.

13.3.3 Application of Anaesthesia and General Medical Complications: Record-Keeping

Local anaesthesia is usually administered with an injection. The dentist must appreciate that receiving an injection may be an uncomfortable event for many people. Therefore, some patients may attribute misunderstood, unexpected or inexplicable events to the giving of an anaesthetic. The following two cases demonstrate this.

■ **Case: Miscarriage**
(Louisiana Court of Appeal, no, 98 Ca 0361 C/W 98 Ca 0362, USA) A female patient approached a dentist complaining of pain. The dentist found a small abscess on a tooth, but advised postponement of the treatment because the patient was pregnant. The pain persisted and the dentist decided on a root canal treatment. The patient was anaesthetised using Citanest. Twelve days later the patient had a miscarriage and blamed this on the administered local anaesthetic. Since the consulted expert stated that the administered dose was defensible for a woman in the second trimester of her pregnancy, the charge was dismissed.

In another example, a patient claimed there was a link between inexplicable pain symptoms and an allergy to the anaesthetic.

13

■ **Case: Allergy**

(Dental Board, 10 May 2001, the Netherlands)
A filling was placed in a patient's tooth under local anaesthesia. Later, pulpitis emerged and the molar was opened under local anaesthesia. After this, the patient returned once again, but this did not result in further treatment. According to the patient, the dentist could not do anything for him, while the dentist claimed this was because the patient had physical complaints and should first be tested for a possible allergy to dental materials – on the patient's record was written 'allergy-nutrition; no dent.restrict. Quickly short of breath'.

Finally, charges were pressed against the dentist for giving anaesthesia twice without establishing whether the patient was allergic to it. The complainant, father of the patient, suggested that the dentist had used the anaesthetic articaine. The complainant had deduced this from the fact that the patient had felt nothing during treatment by the accused dentist and that the patient had felt pain during treatment by another dentist under prilocaine in combination with laser acupuncture. The accused dentist claimed to have used prilocaine and the disciplinary court had no reason to doubt this. The disciplinary court deliberated that it was highly unlikely that an allergic reaction to the anaesthetic had occurred that had led to a pulpitis and dismissed the charge.

Probably, the above case would have been judged in the same way in most other countries.

These cases show that good record-keeping is extremely important. Especially with special patients such as pregnant women and patients with an allergy or another systemic disorder, it is incredibly important to record in the file which anaesthetic has been used and what dosage has been given. It seems that the dentist in the allergy case had a narrow escape. The disciplinary court took for granted that the dentist had used prilocaine and not articaine. The dentist in this case was treated very generously. In the United States, however, several dentists have been sentenced because they did not record in their files the type and dosage of the anaesthetic or a recent medical history.

In the above cases, it was assumed that there was no connection between the local anaesthetic and the medical complaints. After administration of a local anaesthetic, however, medical problems may occur where a direct connection could be assumed between the anaesthesia and the problem.

■ **Case: Overdose**

(Colorado State Board of Dental Examiners, USA)
A dentist extracted seven primary teeth in a child. For the anaesthesia, he used one cartridge of Citanest Plain and three cartridges of Citanest Forte. During the treatment the child

suffered convulsions which subsided after a while, but the child remained unconsciousness for some time. The dental board assumed that this temporary unconsciousness had been caused by the high dose of local anaesthetic. The maximum dose for a patient of this weight was 180.4 mg prilocaine, while the dentist had administered a total of 288 mg. Charges were pressed against the dentist and considered well-founded.

Aside from the anaesthetic, systemic complications may also arise from the added vasoconstrictor.

■   **Case: Brain Haemorrhage After Local Anaesthesia**
(Washington supp court, 28 Wn App 50, USA)
A patient approached his dentist for a wisdom tooth extraction. The previous day, the patient had suffered from such a severe headache; it had felt like his head would explode. The patient was unaware that he was suffering from hypertension and this had never been diagnosed. At the dentist's office, he completed a written medical history, after which the dentist gave him an adrenaline-containing local anaesthetic. After the extraction, the patient became unwell. The following day, his condition deteriorated and a brain haemorrhage or brain infarction was diagnosed. The patient became disabled and died some time later. The dentist was summoned, partly because he had not verified if the patient suffered from hypertension. An expert stated that neglecting to measure the patient's blood pressure went against good care practice in that region at that time. Furthermore, it was considered significant that a textbook warned against the use of adrenaline in patients with hypertension and that the dentist chose not to perform the rather simple blood pressure measurement. One of the judges, however, held the opinion (a concurring opinion) that the statement of the expert did not clarify whether in such cases a dentist should ask if a patient is suffering from hypertension or whether the dentist should measure the patient's blood pressure anyway.

From a dental perspective, some questions can be raised concerning this case, for example, whether there was a clear relation between the vasoconstrictor and the brain haemorrhage. Stress could also have played a role, such as in a similar case in Texas (Court of Appeals Fifth District of Texas, White v Presnall), or it may have been a case of an intravasal injection. One may also wonder whether the expert was perhaps discussing too much retrospectively, for almost all systemic complications after extractions can be avoided if the dentist not only takes an adequate medical history but also consults the patient's general physician or specialist or performs a basic physical examination himself or herself. However, it is not likely that this can be expected of a well-practising dentist, since this would create an unworkable situation. What can be learnt from this case is that, when choosing the local anaesthetic and vasoconstrictor, the dentist should always realise the consequences of this choice for the respective patient. The choice of a specific anaesthetic must be based on a recent medical history that is recorded in the patient's file, if the dentist is wise.

13.3.4   Insufficient Caution During Injection

Occasionally a dentist may be charged for not having exercised enough caution while giving anaesthesia so that a needle breaks, or if he/she did not use a sterile needle.

- **Case: Assistant Pricked First and Then the Patient**

(Court of Special Appeals of Maryland, USA)
A child required a root canal treatment and an extraction. Because the child was wriggling, the dental assistant held the child steady. When giving the anaesthesia, the dentist first inadvertently pricked the assistant and then used the same needle for the patient. The next day, the dentist asked the mother to have the child tested for hepatitis. According to the dentist, the patient was pricked first and then the assistant. The mother phoned the dental assistant who said the opposite had been the case. Eventually an article appeared in a local paper, which attracted the attention of the dental board. On the basis of this incident and other complaints, the dentist's licence was revoked.

Nowadays, local anaesthesia is administered with disposable needles and cartridges. Cases where a needle and cartridge are used for two different people are extremely rare. This does not alter the fact that a dentist should realise that mistakes can be made during the administration of local anaesthesia. For this reason, dentists should give serious consideration to how to minimise complaints about the use of local anaesthesia.

13.4   Avoiding Legal Problems in the Use of Local Anaesthesia

Dentists can avoid many juridical problems by some preventative measures:

- The dentist must be aware of his or her duties, particularly the duty to provide information.
- Without adequate history taking, recorded on the patient's file, any defence will fail.
- If there is any doubt whether anaesthesia is possible and, if so, under which conditions it may be performed, it is sensible to consult the patient's general physician or an oral surgeon.

- If a dentist consults colleagues or takes special precautionary measures, it is wise to note this in the patient's file.
- The burden of the treatment must be as low as possible, especially for medically compromised patients. This may mean that the treatment is performed in more than one session but also that a treatment may be postponed.
- If the dentist is not legally obliged to record every use of anaesthesia in the file, it is advised that the dentist notes in the file when he or she finds it necessary to use another anaesthetic to the usual one.

If the country where the dentist works allows the delegation of the administration of anaesthesia, the following points should be considered:

- The dentist must be aware of the conditions under which this is permissible. Dentists must be convinced themselves that the person they delegate the anaesthesia to has the necessary skills.
- There must be a clear protocol for the administration of anaesthesia, especially to patients at risk, and the procedure in case of complications.
- It is advisable only to delegate if a dentist or doctor can be at the scene very quickly in case of complications. This is automatically the case in jurisdictions where supervision is a prerequisite. In that case the dentist is legally obliged to be at the scene.

Naturally, these guidelines cannot guarantee absolute protection from complaints concerning the use of anaesthesia. However, legal problems are hopefully reduced by them.

13

Further Reading

1. Brands WG. The standard for the duty to inform patients about risks: from the responsible dentist to the reasonable patient. Br Dent J. 2006;201: 207–10.
2. Cohen TH. Punitive damage awards in large counties 2001. US Department of Justice. NCJ 208445; 2005.
3. Loomer PM, Perry DA. Computer-controlled delivery versus syringe delivery of local anesthetic injections for therapeutic scaling and root planing. JADA. 2004;135:358–65.
4. Orr DL, Curtis WJ. Obtaining written informed consent for the administration of local anesthetic in dentistry. JADA. 2005;136:1568–70.
5. Pogrel MA, Schmidt BL, Sambajon V, Jordan RCK. Lingual nerve damage due to inferior alveolar nerve blocks. JADA. 2003;134:195–8.
6. Van Dam B, Bruers J. Permanent sensitivity disorders in patients. Ned Tandartsenbl. 2004;59(16):36–7.

Service Part

© Springer International Publishing Switzerland 2017
J.A. Baart, H.S. Brand (eds.), *Local Anesthesia in Dentistry*, DOI 10.1007/978-3-319-43705-7

Index

CPI Antony Rowe
Eastbourne, UK
September 16, 2019